Praise for
Never Say Diet

"More than 90 percent of my patients gain back most of the weight they lose. Why so little success? The simple answer is that the average person can't stay on a diet permanently. But *this* program is different. It is not a diet but a complete lifestyle, thought-process, and physiological transformation. The change comes from within, helping to make you a better person...not just a thinner person."

—BARRY S. ROSS, MD, Tamarac, Florida

"*Never Say Diet* provides a systematic approach to living a healthier, more balanced life. The food list that Chantel Hobbs presents is nutritious and, most important, enjoyable. *Never Say Diet* proves that fad diets don't work and cannot substitute for creating a lifestyle that leads to attaining your goals."

—LON BEN-ASHER, MS, LD/N, registered dietitian,
North Shore Medical Center, Miami, Florida

"The importance of Chantel's story can't be calculated in terms of burned calories or lost pounds, and it's not her dramatic weight loss that makes her such a special person. It's her willingness to credit God's ability to totally transform lives. She reminds us that lasting change has to happen on the inside before it can happen on the outside and that this change is within reach of anyone who's willing to seize it."

—BOB COY, pastor of Calvary Chapel, Fort Lauderdale, Florida

"You might be able to lose a few pounds with a crash diet, but it's temporary. That's why diets don't work for people who need to lose a lot of weight. Instead of going on a diet, you need to make a lifestyle change. In fact, you must undergo a 'brain change.' *Never Say Diet* delivers just that."

—JOSEPH TEDESCO, DPT, ATC, CSCS, physical therapist,
Elite Physical Therapy, Charlotte, North Carolina

Never Say Diet

Never Say Diet

Make
five decisions
and **break** the fat habit
for good

Chantel Hobbs

with Rowan Jacobsen

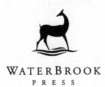

WATERBROOK
PRESS

NEVER SAY DIET
PUBLISHED BY WATERBROOK PRESS
12265 Oracle Boulevard, Suite 200
Colorado Springs, Colorado 80921
A division of Random House Inc.

This book is not intended as a substitute for the advice and care of your physician, and as with
any other fitness, diet, or nutrition plan, you should use proper discretion, in consultation with
your physician, in utilizing the information presented. The author and the publisher expressly
disclaim responsibility for any adverse effects that may result from the use or application of the
information contained in this book.

ISBN 978-1-4000-7449-5

Library of Congress Cataloging-in-Publication Data
Hobbs, Chantel.
  Never say diet : make five decisions and break the fat habit for good / Chantel Hobbs ; with
Rowan Jacobsen. — 1st ed.
      p. cm.
  ISBN 978-1-4000-7449-5
  1. Weight loss. 2. Physical fitness. I. Jacobsen, Rowan. II. Title.
  RM222.2.H573 2007
  613.2'5—dc22

                                    2007035345

Printed in the United States of America
2007—First Edition

10 9 8 7 6 5 4 3 2 1

To the love of my life, Keith,
and our children, Ashley, Kayla, Jake, and Luke.
Your constant encouragement gives me the motivation
to want to be better each day.
I am a blessed woman.

Contents

PART I: Decide

PART II: Act

PART III: Live

Foreword

Right now in the United States, 60 percent of adults are overweight, and a full 30 percent are obese. Several studies have identified a link between obesity and a shortened life span. As a gastroenterologist, I am deeply concerned.

I regularly discuss the importance of exercise and proper nutrition with my patients. Yet it simply does not seem to sink in. Why? Perhaps it's because fad diets and weight-loss centers compete for our attention, and we think going on a diet is the answer. However, it cannot be the best answer, since we still have an extremely difficult time losing weight.

I am sure you know all about the yo-yo experience of dieting. That was me for eighteen years. Finally, through education, personal experience, and outside help, I learned how to keep the unwanted pounds off. About three years ago, as part of my exercise routine, I took a Spinning class taught by an extremely motivated instructor. My ears perked up as I heard phrases such as "Be the best you can be!" I learned about endurance training, peak heart rate, anaerobic threshold, and interval training. I'd certainly never taken a class like this one; it was as if we were being taught by a physiologist! The instructor, of course, was Chantel Hobbs, the author of this book.

I had never met anyone as knowledgeable about nutrition and exercise physiology as Chantel. Now, as I finish reading her marvelous work, *Never Say Diet*, I know this is what America needs. It is what I need in my own armamentarium against obesity. This book is truly inspirational.

This is *not* a new diet or a fitness fad but a real lifestyle and psychological change. The Brain Change is the integral part of the plan, and I am a true believer in it. After reading Chantel's success story, I realized that part of my own continued success has been founded on her principles.

Motivation and unconditional commitment are the cornerstones of any exercise and nutrition program. However, much more is involved. Chantel will show you how to make the right choices. She also explains why you should not be afraid of self-sacrifice. Many diet plans offer temporary success, yet they are missing the psychology and physiology behind permanent life change. It is Chantel's concept of changing the way you think and feel emotionally about food that I find so enlightening.

As you read this book, you will notice that Chantel is convinced we are being scammed by the diet industry. But are we really? I would let statistics from my own medical practice speak for themselves. More than 90 percent of my patients gain back most of the weight they lose on any diet program. Why so little success? The simple answer is that the average person can't stay on a diet permanently. After reading *Never Say Diet*, you will understand why *this* program is different. It is not a diet but a complete lifestyle, thought-process, and physiological transformation. The change comes from within, helping to make you a better person…not just a thinner person.

I wholeheartedly support Chantel's five-phase plan. The cardio and strength training are ideal for all comers, including those who have been involved in other exercise programs and those who have never set foot in a gym. *Never Say Diet* will educate you about body metabolism, calories, fitness for the heart, and how strength training increases metabolic rate. Once you have educated yourself and committed to Chantel's five Brain Change decisions, *Never Say Diet* offers a fantastic exercise program. I do recommend that everyone see their health-care professional for a complete physical exam, including blood work, prior to starting any new program.

We all are striving to be fit and look our best. *Never Say Diet* will help you do just that. In addition, it offers you the chance to achieve a sense of well-being, satisfaction, and long-term health. Read and enjoy.

Barry S. Ross, MD

Tamarac, Florida

Board certified in gastroenterology and internal medicine

Acknowledgments

There are many people who have had a meaningful part in making this book more than just a dream. My parents, Jerry and Sherry, have continued to show me that God is my refuge and that having a fun and passion-filled life is a choice. My in-laws, Ken and Linda, have always made me feel more like a daughter than their son's wife. To my loving and incredibly supportive extended family—there are so many to mention: you are always appreciated. You are proof of God's great sense of humor; He placed each of you in my life.

To my closest friends, Judi Califano and LeeAnn Hansen: I don't know how you could have kept listening during all the hours of my rambling on and on about what I ate and how much I worked out and how Spinning is the greatest invention on the planet. But you always did. Thanks, Jenna Ingraham, for hearing me out when I needed it most. I am so thankful for all my amazing friends. You make me laugh on a regular basis and offer constant encouragement.

I am thankful that my pastor, Bob Coy, has a mission "until the whole world hears." Also that he introduced me to Lou Taylor. Thanks, Lou, for sending me to Chip MacGregor. To my literary agent, Chip: thanks for believing that my story needed to be shared. Thank you also, Rowan Jacobsen, for giving this book your guidance and insight and for listening to my riffs for hours without complaint. To Ron Lee, my editor at WaterBrook Press: your great enthusiasm for this project is more than I could have ever asked for. To the entire WaterBrook team: thanks for your genuine interest in making *Never Say Diet* a reality and for "getting" my excitement and supporting my mission in every way! You are all awesome to work with.

To Joe Tedesco: I appreciate how you jumped in and helped design the strength-training program for the book. Your motivation to get people moving is contagious. Rock on!

To Greg Howard: you are an awesome photographer, and your wife, Ashleigh, complements you perfectly. (greghowardthephotographer.com)

To Dr. Linda Green and John and Yvonne Vasquez: your real-estate investment ended up being much, much more. Having a place of solitude to write has meant more than these pages could ever say. Your generosity is an example of knowing exactly where everything we have comes from.

I want to also thank Lisa Krause for being a part of our family and for loving my kids throughout the years.

I thank God for loving me despite all my flaws and for showing me throughout my life that I can't do anything well without Him.

Finally, along the way I have met countless people who know they can be living a better life and are struggling each day to make that happen. To my clients and my readers, I say, "Listen to my story and believe that you can stay the course. This is possible. Dare to be remarkable. *You* are my constant inspiration!"

Say Good-Bye to Your Excuses

Believe it or not, it is still difficult for me to say the words "I once weighed nearly 350 pounds." Not because I'm ashamed of the person I was, but because I no longer define myself—or others—by weight.

For most of my life, I focused on the number that appeared on the scale and how I appeared in the mirror. Winning my weight war was not quick or easy. Being overweight is a personal battle that makes you feel insecure and weak. Trust me, I tried diets and fads and trendy weight-loss programs, but I kept repeating the same cycle of losing and regaining. Simply put, diets don't work. And it's not always the program that's at fault. If you have tried—and failed—to lose weight and keep it off, the reason you continue to struggle lies in your approach.

I'll bet I've used every excuse you've ever thought of, maybe even several that you haven't. There are plenty of excuses to go around. In fact, at the end of this introduction, I'll list the top twenty excuses I have either used or heard.

You must get beyond all of them. Your only hope for success is to decide not to allow *anything* to stand in your way.

Why do we allow our excuses to control our lives and damage our health and ultimate happiness? I could write a book about self-doubt, denial, and self-hatred. That's where I lived for many years. But I finally reached the point where I was done with living that way. Success began after I made some hard decisions, and I will show you how to make the same decisions so you can tell your own success story.

NEVER SAY DIET AGAIN!

If you are ready to get serious about claiming optimal health and fitness, you are about to begin a life-altering journey. You can achieve much more than you ever dreamed. I know this because it happened to me. I was the woman who could barely squeeze into a seat at the movies and had to stop and rest while walking around Disney World with my kids. Today I'm a marathon runner. I don't have anything special inside me that you don't have. I just got tired of disappointment.

If my story doesn't make you believe in yourself again, then perhaps nothing will. This is your time to start becoming the best you can be, to accept the challenge, and to make a personal commitment to *never say diet* again. It will require discipline and hard work, but the return is greater than you can imagine: a permanent life change. This time you will break the fat habit for good!

Over a period of nearly two years, I lost 200 pounds and got a job as a Spinning instructor. I later started running marathons, and I now work as a personal trainer and life coach. I've seen a great variety of people change their lives by doing the same things I did. In this book I'll show you how to lose weight and keep it off—whether it's 15 pounds or 50 or 150. But much more important than that, I'll show you how to change your life for good. You can reclaim your health and achieve fitness and do it all while juggling the responsibilities of everyday life. Having a demanding job, being a wife and mother, or facing special challenges is no reason to sacrifice your well-being. *Never Say Diet* works in the midst of real life. We will walk through the program together, and you will begin a new life course.

We've all heard that to lose weight long term, you must have a lifestyle change. But that advice is incomplete. To achieve any life change, you must first experience a Brain Change. The good news is that it can happen in a moment, immediately, even though getting weight off takes time. Truthfully, if you don't first change your brain, you will almost certainly fail to permanently change anything in your life. Before you can retrain your body, you must first retrain the way you think about the solutions.

This is not an ordinary fitness book, because it's not simply a recipe for losing weight. Neither is it about physical beauty. The goal is health, fitness, and choosing to live a life of passion and achievement, with no more regret. Therefore, being the best you can be each day is your primary focus. Once you make the Five Decisions and accomplish your Brain Change, you will discover that you automatically choose every day to do what it takes to live this new, exciting, and fulfilling life.

Along with the mental techniques that will get you started and keep you focused, you will learn how to make the best food choices and how to put a realistic system in place for regular exercise. Though I designed my own program when I lost 200 pounds, in this book I have worked closely with experts to make sure the program is as effective as possible for everyone. The nutrition portion is endorsed by Lon Ben-Asher, MS, RD, a clinical dietitian. The cardio and strength-training portion is one I designed with Dr. Joe Tedesco, a certified athletic trainer and physical therapist with a doctorate from Duke University. A medical doctor, Barry Ross, lent his expertise as well, to assure the soundness of the *Never Say Diet* approach. Still, you should consult your personal physician before beginning this or any other nutrition, exercise, and fitness program.

I am blessed to be able to share my story with you. As you begin to make a permanent life change, you can look forward to a lot of fun and the excitement of finding out what it feels like to believe in yourself and your abilities. You will break the barriers that have held you back for too long. Be done with disappointment, and dare to be remarkable!

— • • ● ● ● • —

The Top Twenty Excuses Why You "Can't" Get Fit

It's important to look at the excuses that have prevented you from succeeding in the past. Having been there for most of my life, I'm more than familiar with the leading reasons why people fail to change. These are the twenty excuses I hear most often, either from new clients or from women I meet who say they admire what I've done but know it could never work for them. I used plenty of these myself before I decided to make a permanent change in my life.

See if you recognize some of these excuses—and if you agree with my reasons why they are lame!

1. *I don't have enough hours in the day.*
   The longer you put off addressing your weight and health issues, the more years of life you lose. The time you invest in exercise is returned with interest in extra years of healthy living.
2. *I can't afford a gym membership.*
   Great news: exercise is still free! This book includes workout options that don't cost a cent.
3. *I don't want to be judged on my outer appearance.*
   Too late. We all are.
4. *I'm addicted to sugar.*
   Good, because with this program you get to eat a lot of fruit—nature's candy.

5. *I don't like to work out.*

   Do you love heart doctors and medication? Do you love looking in the mirror and hating yourself?

6. *I don't think this is the right timing.*

   Would it be better to wait until after your next nervous breakdown?

7. *I'm too old to do this.*

   You're still breathing on your own. The older you are, the more you *need* to do this.

8. *I just want to use diet pills.*

   If there were any that worked, don't you think Oprah would have done a show about them already?

9. *I'll get started as soon as I find a partner to do this with.*

   Right, so that when your partner lets you down, it won't be your fault.

10. *I have too much weight to lose.*

    That excuse kept me from getting started for years. Don't think about what you have to lose. You have too much to *gain* not to start today.

11. *I can't stand being hungry when I try to diet.*

    Your body has not been truly hungry in years. You need to retrain your body to know what it needs.

12. *Can't I just get lipo instead?*

    Why use a short-term patch job when you haven't fixed the problem—unless you can afford to keep a plastic surgeon on retainer?

13. *I have the fat gene.*

    Yeah, so do I.

14. *I always fail.*

    Nobody can maintain that perfect record forever. Whether you think you can or think you can't, you're right!

15. Isn't healthy food expensive?

Doctor visits are expensive. Lipitor prescriptions are expensive. Natural foods like eggs, apples, greens, and oatmeal are cheap.

16. I need to lose this weight as fast as possible.

Studies show that rapid weight loss leads to subsequent rapid weight gain. Put the time in to learn how to make weight loss last forever.

17. I hate paying attention to calories.

Bad news! Losing weight requires math. But we'll keep it like kindergarten, not calculus.

18. I don't want to look like a bodybuilder.

The workouts in this program are designed to make you lean and fit, not bulky.

19. I might give this a shot. I have nothing to lose.

Wrong attitude. You've already got one foot out the door. When you're ready to commit 100 percent to success, come back.

20. I have negative people around me.

Good. Let me bring them to my family reunion! They'll feel right at home.

• • • ● • • •

PART ONE

• • • • • •

Decide

Chapter 1

The Night That Changed My Life

How to Choose to Do the Best Job of Living

I t should have been a scene of American family bliss. A Sunday afternoon in our home on a beautiful fall day in South Florida. My husband, Keith, was watching the Dolphins game in the living room with some friends. He'd waited all week for this. Our girls, six-year-old Ashley and four-year-old Kayla, were helping me in the kitchen. Well, kind of. Our six-month-old, Jake, was jumping and laughing in his Jolly Jumper. I was baking Vanishing Oatmeal Raisin Cookies, our favorite, and everybody could smell the cinnamon and butter and couldn't wait for the cookies to come out of the oven. Especially me.

As I worked in the kitchen, I could hear the football game coming from the living room. The announcers were talking about a player who had arrived at training camp completely out of shape. He was six foot four and weighed 320 pounds. "That is a big boy," they said. "Wow! He is *huge*."

"Would you look at that guy," I heard my husband say with disgust. "I can't believe he got so fat! What a lazy bum."

Those words cut me to the heart. I had created a happy home, with a happy husband and happy kids. But at that moment I wanted to die, because I outweighed that player by at least 10 pounds. I was bigger than anyone playing for the Miami Dolphins. And I knew I was anything but lazy.

I pulled the cookies out of the oven and felt nauseous. I was pathetic. I'd been overweight my entire adult life, but I was bigger than I had ever been. I was miserable but doing an excellent job of faking out everyone who knew me. I was five foot nine and weighed 330 pounds, maybe more. I didn't know for sure because it had been months since I'd dared to step on a scale. Besides, the only one in the house was a conveniently inaccurate discount-store model with a wheel underneath that calibrated the scale. I had adjusted it to register the lowest weight possible. I was in denial, but I was also without hope. It was the autumn of 2000. I was twenty-eight years old and was starting to believe I would never live a long and fulfilled life. Not this way.

If an angel had landed on my shoulder and whispered in my ear that, in less than two years, Oprah Winfrey would have me on her show to tell a feel-good weight-loss story, I'd have sent that angel packing and gone back to my cookies. I wasn't Oprah material. And there was absolutely nothing feel-good about my life. Call me when you want a feel-bad story. That was me.

If that angel had whispered that I would one day run a marathon, I'd have checked him in to an insane asylum. I couldn't run around the block. Even in high school I hadn't been able to run the required twenty-minute mile. My knees hurt all the time. I was morbidly obese—a term that I knew meant an early death. If one thing was clear about my life in the fall of 2000, it was that I could never, ever run a marathon.

But I did. I finished my first one in 2005 and after that ran four more—in less than a year. I went from weighing nearly 350 pounds to less than 150 pounds. And I have appeared on *Oprah* and *Good Morning America* and the cover of *People* magazine as one of America's great weight-loss successes. Getting fit wasn't easy—there was plenty of pain, deprivation, tears, and hunger along the way. It was the hardest thing I've ever done, and I won't try to sugarcoat any of that. But, honestly, I didn't give myself a choice. Once I made the unconditional decision that I was going to lose weight and get healthy, nothing could stop me. And nothing will stop you if you make the Five Decisions to break the fat habit for good. That's a guarantee.

Here is the secret I learned—the same secret I want to share with you. I realized I had to change my mind before I could change my body, my health, and my life. I discovered the Five Decisions, which brought about an unconditional commitment to getting healthy and fit. Once I started, I treated it like a job so that no matter what else was going on in my life, I did what I had to do to achieve daily goals, weekly goals, monthly goals, and eventually the target weight and fitness that I desired. After making the Five Decisions, getting fit was a matter of showing up for work each day. The process developed from the inside out, which was a new concept for me.

FIRST, YOU CHANGE YOUR MIND

People constantly ask me how I lost 200 pounds and started running marathons. When I explain that it took several years to achieve those goals, they wonder how I was able to stick to the plan when so many others can't. I ask myself the same question. I had failed plenty of times before. I'd tried a few diets and failed, including a bit of foolishness called the chocolate-wafer diet, which I'll tell you about later. I'd resolved so many times not to eat the entire package of Oreos, without success. So how did I lose all that weight and keep it off—reclaiming my health and gaining a new life in the process?

Here's the simple answer: my brain changed. I decided to first become a different person in my mind and then learned patience as my body followed. My success wasn't measured only by a declining number on a scale; it was much deeper. I had to change on the inside. I needed to change my mind before I could change my body.

It will work the same way for you. First you must get to the right place in your head, and then you can create the lifestyle to go along with that. Your body reflects your daily choices, so stop confusing it by the way you think.

The mistake so many people make is to focus on weight loss and how long it will take. In fact, the multibillion-dollar diet industry banks on people thinking this way. Don't get stuck in the weight loss–weight gain cycle. What you should focus on is the person you want to be. Set your sights *very* high, and keep your commitment level *even higher.*

In this book I'll explain how I did that. I went from being someone who weighed more than a Miami Dolphins lineman to someone who is strong and trim and can run twenty-six miles. I went from a state of hopelessness to a life of incredible confidence. And I want to help you achieve something great in your life. If you change your mind before attempting to change your body, you can do this.

HITTING ROCK BOTTOM

While I was learning how to lose weight and regain my health, I faced setback after setback. My husband lost his job, and my mother was diagnosed with cancer—and those were only two of the crises that came along. Changing your life will never be easy, and that's why in order to succeed, you first need to be ready to succeed. It's a choice you make.

In the fall of 2000, when I was baking cookies and overhearing my husband's criticism of an overweight NFL lineman, I fell into despair. I realized my life was out of control and I was headed for an early grave if I didn't change. But even then, I wasn't yet ready to make the commitment that was necessary to change my life. The truth is, on that dark day I still wasn't miserable enough to change.

I hit rock bottom about six months later. I was at my heaviest ever—349 pounds, I think. Though I was still mostly in denial, I was starting to see myself clearly, and I hated what I saw. I'd look in the mirror and say, "You are pitiful! How could you have let this happen?"

My appearance started to affect my family life. We live in South Florida, where every weekend is a pool party. My daughters were young, but they were being invited to a few parties, and I was horribly uncomfortable in a bathing suit. I knew it wouldn't be long before my girls would be embarrassed by their mother, and that made me want to cry. It *did* make me cry. But that was the least of it. I was more worried that their mom would die young. I'd seen fat people, and I'd seen old people, but rarely had I seen fat, old people. If I couldn't change for myself, maybe I could do it for my kids.

One night I was driving home alone from an event at church. I felt trapped in despair. At age twenty-nine, my body felt old. I had recently had an emergency gallbladder operation, and the doctor had told me he was afraid to cut through all my layers of fat because of the risk of infection. Imagine being worried about your diseased gallbladder and experiencing anxiety about surgery. And then you learn that your weight problem makes you more prone to infection.

That night in the car I felt like the most pathetic person who had ever lived. I believed that God had made me and put me on earth for a purpose, and I was not living the life He intended for me. I knew I had to change.

As I drove, drowning in self-pity, I began to envision what my life would be if I weren't fat. I thought of all the things I could do—even simple things, such as walking down an airplane aisle without having to turn sideways. I'd be able to board a flight without getting fearful stares from people hoping I wouldn't sit next to them. And there were deeper things, such as being able to go down a slide at a playground with my kids. And I wanted never again to feel as if I was embarrassing my husband when he introduced me to business associates. I was tired of feeling prejudged by every server in every restaurant for what I ordered. I wanted to be able to shop in the same clothing stores as all my friends.

I wanted a normal life.

As I drove home from church, I came to the realization that I absolutely could not go on with my life as it was. I pulled over, sobbing. In total despair I cried out to God. I remember every word. "This is it!" I said. "I can't live like this anymore. I'm done. I give all this pain to You. I surrender this battle. I need You to take over and give me a plan. Otherwise, I don't want to live anymore."

Almost immediately a sense of inner peace filled me, and I calmed down. I had gone to church all my life and had a relationship with God, but I had certainly never felt anything like that before. The peace was real, and in my mind I heard from God. I clearly heard these words: *You are not being the best you can be.* It wasn't a booming voice like in a movie, but it also wasn't a voice coming from me. The words were a jolt to my soul. And that moment would change my life forever.

Again, with crystal clarity, I "heard" a whisper: *You are not being the best you can be.* And for the first time in my life, I understood that this was a choice. I could choose to be the best I could be or not. We all have the same choice. We can't choose our natural talents or what opportunities life is going to throw our way, but we can choose to do this one thing: we can do the best job of living that we are capable of. After praying alone in my car, I knew I could do better.

THE CHOICE IS YOURS

No matter how overweight and out of shape we are, our bodies and minds are capable of much more than we think. No matter what battles we face in life, we can have victory. The amazing thing is that so many of us choose not to. I know this is true because I was as guilty as anyone. For years I'd made poor choices and come up with excuses for why I really didn't have a choice at all. I was big boned. I let myself overeat because I was pregnant. I skipped exercise because I didn't have the time. I was too far gone to ever recover. I told myself whatever it took to hide the truth that I was not doing the best job of living.

I was also being scammed by the diet industry. We all have been taken in by the hype. "We'll give you your eating points," the industry tells us, "and let you spend them on any food you want. And we'll love you when you get on that scale, whether you've lost weight or not. We'll keep hugging you for the next twenty-three years if need be." Counting my points was not going to save me. Choosing the right frozen entrée and having it delivered to my home for the next two years was not going to save me. I didn't need the unconditional love of strangers; I needed unconditional commitment from myself.

I was also scammed by the "fat gene" scientists who insisted that my weight problem was out of my hands. They were wrong; it *was* in my hands. *Chantel,* I told myself, *this is not cancer.* I knew, because my mother had leukemia, and I had spent more tearful nights than I could count praying for her recovery—something I couldn't do anything about. I prayed that chemotherapy would work and that God would heal her. But I realized that I'd been thinking of my obesity in the same way, as an illness. I'd even been told by experts that drastic surgery might be my only option. But that was another lie. The way I lived my life and how I contributed to my health were completely in my hands.

Every one of us knows what we should do, but we don't always do it.

Instead, we pretend it's out of our control. We take the easy way out and let ourselves down. Gaining weight doesn't come about by accident, and it's not forced on us. We gain weight through a series of poor choices made on a regular basis over a long period of time.

> *We gain weight through a series of poor choices made on a regular basis over a long period of time.*

The same process holds true for achieving a goal related to your health and fitness. Whether it's weight loss, athletic accomplishment, or any other personal or business goal, you achieve what you seek by learning to make the right choices and not being scared of self-sacrifice. I began wondering what my life would be like and what I would be capable of if I simply started being the best me I could.

It was time to find out.

After hearing God tell me, *You are not being the best you can be,* I made my decision, and I said it out loud: "I can do this. I *will* do this." I repeated it, and I meant it. At that moment by the side of Cypress Creek Road, my life turned around.

DO IT, THEN TALK

Having made the commitment, I knew I was going to change my life, but I didn't have a specific plan. I knew I'd have to start exercising, no matter how much I dreaded it. I knew I would have to change the way I ate, and I would need to learn more about nutrition. And to become a different person, I knew I would have to start thinking like the person I wanted to be and not the person I had allowed myself to become. I didn't know how I was going to do all this, but I knew I would have God by my side. He might not make it easy, but He'd give me the strength to do everything that was needed.

When I got home that night, Keith was already in bed. He had never criticized my weight, for which I was incredibly grateful, but I knew how he must have felt. I looked into my husband's eyes, told him that God had spoken to me in the car, and announced that the next morning I would begin losing weight and getting healthy. (I even mentioned that one day I would write a book to reach others in my situation.) I made it clear that I was totally committed to being the best I could be.

Keith smiled at me and quoted one of his favorite sources of inspiration, the self-made billionaire Art Williams: "Do it, then talk."

He was right. I shut up. Keith fell asleep, but I had a burning passion that kept me awake that night and has kept me up many nights since. Making the unconditional decision to change—the complete commitment with no turning back—had to be followed by *action*. First you change your mind. But to change your body and your life, you have to get moving. You have to do things and do them differently from the past. *Do it*. How incredibly simple—yet how long it had taken me to get to a place where I could see that clearly. Getting fit and accomplishing my dreams was simply a matter of choosing to do it, following through every single day, and understanding that failure was not an option. I could do it. I *would* do it.

And I did.

Keep reading, and you'll find out how to change your life through five crucial decisions. The Five Decisions change your brain, giving you a new way of thinking about yourself, your life, your health, and your future. As long as you keep thinking the same way you always have, you will keep doing the things you have always done—including the unhealthy habits you have developed.

Join me in the next chapter as we explore the past—including all the influences that worked together to bring us to where we are today. Understanding the messages that influence our self-perception and the way we respond to obstacles enables us to make the new decisions that are necessary for permanent change.

• • • • • •

What Do You Want to Change, and Why?

As you prepare to make the mental changes that will lead to permanent life change, think through the reasons you want to change. What is motivating your desire to lose weight and reclaim your health? Use the questions that follow to think in detail about your life, your goals for the future, and what you're willing to do to make this happen finally and forever.

1. Beyond losing weight, what do you most want to change about your life?

2. Are you willing to do whatever it takes to see certain areas of your life undergo radical change? If you're not yet willing, what is holding you back?

3. When in your life have you felt the most hopeless? Are you now ready to move past those scars and never look back?

4. When you gained weight in the past, what factors caused you to lose your focus on health?

5. Identify three reasons or influences from the past that convinced you that you couldn't achieve permanent life change. After considering these reasons, can you now admit they were merely excuses?

6. Think about the necessity of changing your mind before you attempt to change your body. Do you agree that lasting change begins on the inside? As you consider being the best you can be, are you ready to work from the inside out?

7. A total life change involves your mind, body, and spirit. Think about the spiritual aspect for a moment. Do you accept the role that faith plays in the process of changing your life for good?

8. When have you been held back by a fear of failure? Write down your biggest fears in this regard. As you face your fears, can you decide to let them go and give your all to permanent life change?

• • • • • • •

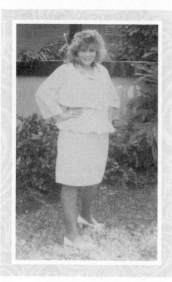

Fourteen and already fighting fat

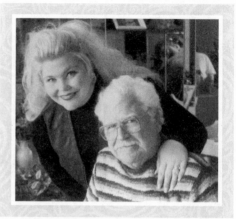

Me with my big hair and my grandfather, Pepa

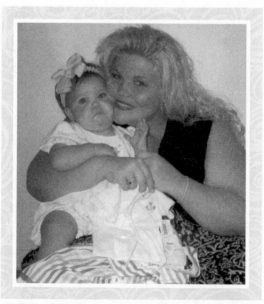

With my daughter Kayla as a toddler. When posing for photos, I had mastered the art of having a child in front of me.

Chapter 2

"You Have Such a Pretty Face"

Facing the Pain of How Others See You

I was in second grade when I first realized I was not like the other little girls. I was sitting in a classroom at one of those hexagonal tables all elementary schools seem to have, and another girl pulled her chair up to mine so we could share crayons. We were both wearing shorts, and the girl asked, "How come your legs are so much bigger than mine?" I looked down and saw that my leg was twice the size of hers. It had never occurred to me that I might be different, but that day it became clear that I was bigger than the other kids. *Wow, am I a fat girl?* When I got home, I weighed myself on my mother's scale. I was only eight years old, and already I weighed 80 pounds.

What did I know about being fat at such a young age? Not much, but I knew it wasn't something that anyone wanted to be. When you're a kid, you don't want to be different in any way, and being bigger meant being laughed at.

All on my own I decided I had to do something. I remember being in a Sunday school class at the Church of the Nazarene in Hollywood, Florida. Just like on other Sundays, the teachers passed out cookies to the kids. They were butter cookies in the shape of little flowers, with a hole in the middle. They came from Winn-Dixie and will be instantly familiar to you if you grew up in the seventies or eighties. I loved cookies, but this time as the teacher passed out five or six to each student, I thought, *I can't have those.* "No thanks," I said, "I'm not gonna have any."

My teacher looked at me. "Why not? You like these cookies."

"I'm on a diet," I said.

"That's silly. Little girls don't go on diets. Here, eat your cookies." She gave me my pile, and I ate it. *How nice. Little girls don't have to go on diets.*

Thus ended my first dieting attempt. I never mentioned the incident to my mother. At eight, I was already fighting a private battle—and I didn't know what to do about it.

Later in second grade, the day before track-and-field day at school, my grandmother took my sister and me shopping. My grandmother didn't have a lot of money, but she loved to treat us by taking us to the Hollywood Fashion Center. We'd visit Jordan Marsh, JCPenney, and Sears, then swing by Fannie Farmer for a chocolate lollipop. On this particular day we were hunting for the perfect outfit for track-and-field day. We searched in every store, but we couldn't find shorts that fit me. They all were too tight. Finally a lady at Sears suggested the girls-plus department. Sure enough, we found several pairs that fit. I was relieved but mad. I didn't know what girls-plus meant, but I knew it wasn't a regular size. *Okay, now I have to get clothes in a special area. There's something wrong with me.*

My grandmother, my mother, and everyone else in my family went out of their way not to make me feel bad about my weight. But still, I felt fat, and I knew it made me different and somehow "less" than other kids.

THE LOVE OF JUNK FOOD

When people see overweight kids, they assume that heaviness runs in the family or that the family feasts on pizza and fried chicken. Neither was true for me. A few of my great aunts were morbidly obese, but my immediate family looked normal. And my mother put a healthy, home-cooked meal on the table every night. After my grandmother died from pancreatic cancer when I was in the third grade, my mom put even more effort into serving healthy food. She read every label and even entered a macrobiotic phase, journeying to nearby farms for fresh brown eggs and goat's milk. We had lentils for dinner at least once a week, and our dessert was often fake hot chocolate made with carob.

People say that if you introduce kids to healthy, natural foods at an early age, that's what they'll like to eat. If only it were that simple. I do think it's important to get kids eating right as early as possible, and I make a big effort with my own kids to instill healthy habits. But for any kid, a carrot cannot compete with a peanut butter cup. I discovered the joys of junk food at an early age, and I just happened to live in a time and place where a resourceful girl could have almost unlimited access to the stuff.

Every day after school I would spend my lunch money on a Slurpee and a Clark Bar at the 7-Eleven. When I put something sweet in my mouth, it tasted so good, and I felt happy. It was that simple. But then I'd swallow, and it was gone, and the happiness would disappear as well, so I needed more junk.

I always wanted to maintain the sugar high. It would be a long time before I discovered a substitute for the happy feeling of sugar, something that would keep me feeling good long after the event was over. Exercise and the pride of accomplishment eventually replaced the sugar high.

But back then I was anything but active. When I was in school, overweight kids didn't play sports. My friends were often busy with cheerleading or softball practice, so I spent my after-school hours indoors watching television and snacking. My parents had started a furniture business, and that took up much of their time. My mom even worked nights as a nurse to pay the bills. She would come home in the morning as we were waking up, give us breakfast, take us to school, sleep a little, then head over to the furniture business to do paperwork. In the afternoon she would drive us home from school and then try to catch up on her rest. My siblings and I had many unsupervised afternoons. There was us, the television, and the convenience store up the block.

I don't blame my parents for my weight issues. They were, and are, incredibly loving. My mom didn't keep junk food around, though she loved to bake. She never could have anticipated that her daughter would develop a fullblown obsession with food.

As a little girl, if something tasted good to me, I wanted more. After I ate the junk food I'd bought with my lunch money, I'd do anything to get more. My little brothers and I would collect soda-pop bottles around the neighborhood. We'd even take things from the house—boxes of index cards, nail-polish remover, my mother's jewelry—pile it in our wagon, and sell it to our neighbors until we had enough cash. Then I'd go to Cumberland Farms for chocolate chip ice cream—a whole pint. Sometimes I sent my brothers because I was embarrassed for the clerk to see me there again. Then I would watch television and eat ice cream, the entire pint, until I felt sick. And before long, it was time for dinner.

I could never understand why I did this. I had a great life. I had a big family, and I was loved. Was boredom a factor? Sure. But I wasn't eating to fill an emotional void. I was eating because I felt good every time I put a spoonful in my mouth.

WHY WE EAT

It's a myth that all fat people eat for emotional reasons. Looking back, I believe I was competitive and compulsive, and I needed an outlet. I think a lot of overweight people are that way. Food just becomes the obsession. It was the eighties, and I was caught in a trap: access to cheap sugar, little supervision, and the discovery of an unhealthy hobby involving food.

I fell in love with sweets. One day a cake became the ultimate prize. I'll never forget going to a school carnival with my aunt Michele. I saw the cakewalk and couldn't believe the selection of cakes to be awarded as prizes. One in particular dazzled me. It was a big, pink, layer cake with Starlight Mints all over it. I entered the cakewalk determined to win but tied with another girl who got to pick before me. Of course she picked the pink cake, leaving me with a pineapple upside-down cake.

"That's mine!" I screamed, pointing at the layer cake. Whatever the girl saw in my eyes, she realized it would be dangerous to come between me and the pink cake, so she gave in. Bursting with pride, I carried it out of the carnival, then almost dropped it. "You better watch out," Aunt Michele said, "or you *will* have an upside-down cake." I laughed. I was intensely happy. I thought I had done something great that day.

I know there are people, like my husband, who aren't wired this way. Sweets start to turn Keith off pretty fast. A few bites and he's done. But for me, the last Swiss Cake Roll tastes every bit as good as the first.

Although my mother had no idea how much junk food I was sneaking, she could see the changes in my body. She tried to talk to me about it, but she'd been thin all her life. What did she know about being overweight? She told me I needed to pay attention to the inner feeling that told me I was full. I thought, *What do you mean? What is "full"? What is "enough"?* For me, full was when I had eaten so much I was ready to throw up.

My mother was a nurse, and when I was ten, she got the idea that I might have a thyroid problem. It made sense, because no one else in the family was overweight. I desperately hoped it was true. If I could get my thyroid fixed, I would become a normal, skinny girl. We went to the hospital to get my blood drawn, and our pastor's wife happened to be working at the reception desk. She asked why we were there, and my mother told her. I was so embarrassed that I wanted to run out of the hospital. (It's still hard for me to talk about the person I was back then. People often judge you if they find out you were ever out of control for any reason.)

I had a weight issue, but I would rather have driven needles under my fingernails than call attention to my weight. By the time I was a teen, my size was a source of incredible misery. At some level, in spite of the size on my clothing labels, I refused to accept it. Though I struggled for years in my attempts to overcome it, I would never, ever have said, "I am a fat person."

But that was a problem. By avoiding the truth, I was making personal change impossible. Today I'm convinced that owning up to our weight problems—and refusing to accept that we have to exist like that—is an essential step toward losing excess weight. In chapter 6, we will look at the Five Decisions we have to make before permanent weight loss is possible. One of the decisions is to stop allowing ourselves an out. As soon as we start to think, *Maybe this is how I was meant to be,* we have lost the weight battle as well as any other battles we face. So don't buy that lie. When I meet overweight women who talk about their latest failed diet attempts, I sense that they are too comfortable with failure. They aren't yet miserable enough to change.

That was never me. My misery became great enough to make me question whether life was worth living that way. But fixing it was a long time in coming.

"You Have Such a Pretty Face"

Before I became too miserable to stay the way I was, I had to endure years of judgment and disappointment. I was ten years old when I first heard the words that would come to symbolize my struggle. My sister and I were sitting on a quilt at a church picnic, playing with Barbie dolls, when my mom introduced us to a new friend of hers. Christy and I looked nothing alike. I was blond and green eyed; she had hazel eyes and dark hair. I was chubby; she was a rail. After my mom introduced us, the friend looked at Christy and said, "Oh, that one is so gorgeous!" Then she looked at me. "And your other daughter *has such a pretty face.*" I can't tell you how many times I heard those words in the years that followed. The woman was trying to compliment me, but she was implying that the rest of me was definitely not gorgeous. I knew exactly what she meant, and it hurt me deeply.

Fast-forward to high school and filling out forms at the end of the year to match students with the superlatives that captured their personality and accomplishments: best student, most likely to succeed, brightest smile, and so on. One category was for best-looking girl. A friend named Vicky announced to the kids sitting around us, "Why don't we change this one to 'prettiest face'? Then we can all write down Chantel." I begged her with all my heart not to, and she dropped it. She meant it sincerely, but if they had written me in, it would have become the class joke, and I knew it. *Please stop talking about me.*

I was twenty-two when I had my first baby, Ashley. After the delivery, the nurse brought her to me. Ashley had flawless skin and big blue eyes. "She has your beautiful face," the nurse told me. I couldn't take it as a compliment, because I knew I weighed more than 300 pounds. *Please, lady, just say she's a beautiful baby. And please, God, don't ever let my daughter know this pain.*

Year after year I kept hearing that I had such a pretty face. It was code for "You could look so much better if you weren't fat."

The worst part was that it was true. I *could* look better. More important, I could *be* better. When I was a kid, I knew I had a lot to offer. I was funny and entertaining. I was friendly. Yet I always felt left out. I was ready to be a good friend, but other girls would go out of their way to exclude me. I wanted to be in style, but Jordache jeans didn't come in my size. I tried my best with fashion, but wearing turned-over socks with pumps and a headband with a bow would never make me look like Madonna. Even my voice coach told me I could hold notes longer if I lost weight. *Gee, thanks. Criticize the one thing people say I'm good at.*

> *When you're overweight,*
> *people never really see you*
> *for yourself, because they've already*
> *marked you as different.*

My weight hampered everything I tried to do, everything I wanted to be. It put me on my own little planet. Most moments throughout the day were spent worrying about potential embarrassment. When you're overweight, people never really see you for yourself, because they've already marked you as different. This adds to your isolation. Others don't see the person inside the fat. And what they can't see, they can't connect with.

I spent the summer before I started high school in fear of the embarrassment that I knew was in store for me. I was stuck in a fat trap and had no clue how to get out. I knew very little about nutrition—though I certainly understood that eating nachos and powdered donuts for lunch was not helping. Neither was avoiding exercise. I would go to extremes not to dress out for PE. I'd rather have failed the class than come out of the locker room wearing shorts.

SEEKING HELP FROM THE DIET INDUSTRY

Between ninth and tenth grade, I asked my mom to take me to a Doctor's Weight Loss Clinic. I had seen the amazing before-and-after photos in the window, and I longed to be one of the success stories. At the clinic, a young guy from my school took a Polaroid of me. I was wearing size 24 teal jeans, and I wanted to die when he told me to step on the scale. I weighed 262 pounds. I was mortified to be on any scale, let alone in front of a cute boy.

The clinic gave me an eating plan, and I stuck to it. By my sweet-sixteen birthday in January 1988, I was down to 199 pounds and feeling good. *Yes, under 200!* I asked my counselor if she thought it would be okay to have a piece of cake at my birthday party. She replied, "A taste to the lips adds inches to the hips." It sounded ridiculous and hurtful. I thought, *I don't need you anymore. I can do this on my own.* I never went back.

Now that I help others with their weight loss, I realize how that counselor destroyed my motivation and willingness to keep up my disciplined eating. She was talking to a girl who had lost 63 pounds and was doing really well, and instead of offering praise and encouragement, she made me feel like a disobedient puppy. If I ate the cake, she'd rub my nose in it.

Lots of diet plans offer temporary success, but they miss the psychology behind permanent life change. For weight loss to last a lifetime, the approach has to fit the realities of life. With the right coaching, a little birthday cake did not need to be the end of my progress. It even could have been a celebration of my impressive accomplishment.

AN OVEREATER'S WARPED PERSPECTIVE

If you struggle with out-of-control food issues like I did, then knowing that you should eat more vegetables and lean protein and that you should exercise regularly are not going to make a difference. To make a change, you first need to understand your warped perspective. In my case I *knew* that losing weight was the long-term solution to my unhappiness. But when you weigh more than 300 pounds, it seems like an impossible goal. I can remember thinking, *Losing the weight will take too long, but eating cake is something I can do right now!* How crazy is that?

Perhaps you have relied on the same lack of logic: "I feel terrible about my weight, so I'm gonna eat to feel better!" When we're desperate, we do what we need to self-medicate.

When I felt hopeless, food was the answer I sought. Occasionally it was potato chips or pizza, but usually I went looking for sweets. I remember having a fight with my husband over something stupid. I headed straight to the bakery at Publix. The first thing I found was a glazed croissant. Croissants, you see, are not fattening enough, so it's nice that they glaze them. I knew one would not give me a good fix, so I bought three—two for then, one for later. Well, you'd be surprised how fast two glazed croissants can disappear while sitting in your car outside a grocery store. A few minutes later I found myself driving and eating the third one. And that solved my original problem. I had forgotten all about the fight with Keith. Now I could focus on hating myself for being a fat cow!

Feeling like a failure, time after time, was exhausting. Not that others would have thought of me as a failure. From high school onward, my solution to my weight problem was to do everything humanly possible to draw attention to something other than my size. I became a classic overcompensator. I came across as cheerful and full of life. Others thought I had amazing confidence.

At age fifteen, I even had my first boyfriend.

My future husband and I met at church, just after I had lost my weight at the Doctor's Weight Loss Clinic. Keith and I became fast friends. We went to church camp together that summer and shared our first kiss. *Wow, a guy who really likes me.* Keith told me I was beautiful and never criticized my weight. We dated throughout high school, and my weight kept creeping up. *Why bother dieting when my boyfriend already thinks I'm beautiful?* At the prom I felt like a fuchsia whale in yards of stuffed satin, but I hid my pain and concentrated on the bright future I hoped we'd have together.

We were engaged in 1992, and I resolved to lose weight for the wedding. The next week I got acquainted with another dimension of the diet industry, a multilevel-marketing program that sold chocolate wafers. I even signed up to be a representative. One day you eat nothing but Metamucil-like chocolate wafers and drink water. The next day you get to eat anything you want. The theory is that you can't possibly eat enough on your free day to make up for what you've skipped on your wafer day. Well, ha ha. It wasn't too hard to schedule my entire life around the days I got to eat. After one month, I weighed 2 pounds more than when I started. End of diet.

That fall a day came that all girls dream of—I got to go shopping for a wedding dress. When I finally found one I liked, I was disappointed that I couldn't try it on. It was a rack size 6. The shop ordered the dress in the largest size it came in, 24, and assured me it would fit. When it arrived, I encountered my worst nightmare: there was a six-inch gap across the back where the zipper failed to close. I was so humiliated. The shop had to order extra fabric and have a seamstress remake my dress. It felt like I was wearing a big, white tent.

Despite my disappointment about my weight, Keith and I had a beautiful wedding day in February, complete with a rainbow. To me, this was a promise from God that my life was getting better. Six months later I became pregnant, and Ashley was born in June 1994.

We were a classic new family: very young and very broke. To alleviate our money worries, I ate. It was always the easiest and cheapest fix for my mood. To be able to stay home with Ashley, I baby-sat some other children. Stuck in the house all day with other people's crying babies, I would eat out of frustration and boredom. I thought about dieting—a lot—but soon I became pregnant again. And there's no point in dieting while you're pregnant, right? I started that pregnancy at 336 pounds.

People who knew me then would have told you that I wasn't embarrassed by my weight. They would have said I was confident and happy. Yet I was living a lie. I was always conscious of my weight, and it cast a shadow over every event in my life. By the time Kayla was born in 1996, my husband had accompanied me to many obstetrician appointments, where I had to step on the dreaded scale. Still Keith had no clue how much I weighed. You wouldn't believe the energy I put into scheming ways to keep my weight a secret. There were a few close calls when I had to hop off the scale as I saw my husband coming, and I had to pray that the nurse wouldn't open my file or casually mention my weight while he was around. Insane.

Years later, after I had made the Five Decisions and had lost about 85 pounds, I was finally ready to let Keith watch me get on a scale. The look on his face was comical as he stared at the number—258 pounds. It wasn't *Wow, honey, you've lost a lot of weight!* It was a look of shock. As he did the math, he realized where I'd started.

BREAKING FREE FROM THE FAT TRAP

When you're caught in the fat trap, you become familiar with the crazy psychology of trying to disguise your size. I always looked neat and put together. I even applied makeup every time I went into labor! I became a master of posing for photos with a baby on my lap to hide my body. I felt that if I could be extraordinary in every other way—dress my daughters in matching headbands and outfits, be a good Christian mom, make my husband's favorite dinner, keep my house spotless, plan elaborate parties for my kids—then maybe people would overlook my obvious defect.

Because I was so unhappy with myself, I had to look to others for praise. But no matter how much praise I received, it couldn't fix the fact that I was always disappointed in myself. I even wondered if God was disappointed in me. Yet I still wasn't willing to accept the fact that I needed to give the pain to Him, that only He could understand and take it away.

Then came the night I was driving home from a church meeting and I heard the message from God: *You are not being the best you can be.* I don't believe those words were meant just for me. I believe they are meant for every person. My light-bulb moment happened when it did because I was finally ready to accept that the way I was living was unacceptable. I was done with my old excuses.

What about you? If you are overweight or burned out in your career or stuck in some other way, don't let yourself off the hook. Make the decision to stop putting off the change you desire. Do something *now.* And don't do it to please anyone else, but do it because you want to live with excitement and passion.

Don't wait another day for your light-bulb moment. You just had it.

Ten Things You Must Understand Before You Can Change

1. Overeating isn't just emotional.

Eating feels good, but that doesn't mean enjoying food is any more of an emotional crutch than enjoying other pleasures in life. Getting a pedicure, having a facial, and hugging your children are meant to make you feel good. Yes, I developed an unhealthy relationship with food. But trying to write it off as a misguided search for love, as some diet books do, was not reality for me. Many of us overeat because certain foods taste really, really good and we can't get enough. Then we end up miserable. It's necessary to identify the emotional issues involved in your struggle with food, but don't use those issues to justify your bad choices.

2. Some of us are rigged differently.

There are people like my mom and my husband who get "full" signals from their brains pretty fast, and they listen to those signals. The third doughnut is unthinkable to them. I was never like that, and I'm confident that most of us who struggle with our weight are rigged differently. Of course, we know that just because we can eat ten doughnuts doesn't mean we should. But it does mean we need to come up with fresh strategies other than the "listen to your body" advice dispensed by naturally thin people.

3. The snares of the fat trap are laid early.

Once a kid is overweight, she is unlikely to play sports or to exercise. And at that point, her odds of getting fit and healthy plummet. As overweight kids get ostracized by society, they become more likely to stay at home to avoid teasing. And that is where the twin temptations of television and snack food await. If that describes your childhood, know that you are going to have to sacrifice your comfort and reconnect with the world. And if the above describes your child, get her active and engaged as soon as possible, and live the example!

4. Society is not going to help.

I don't need to say "supersize" to convince you that eating establishments will hand you all the ice cream, pastries, and sodas you want, all the way to the grave. If you're ready to change your ways, realize that you'll have to start on the inside. Help will not come from society.

5. Lying to yourself doesn't help.

I rigged my scale to read a few pounds low and even stayed away from the scale for months on end. Who was that helping? I applied perfect makeup and wore stylish shoes in hopes that people wouldn't notice I was 200 pounds overweight. I unintentionally did everything I could to prolong my misery. Living that way just deepened the unhappiness and the denial. If you're ready to change, get ready to tell yourself the truth.

6. Understanding nutrition will help.

My problems with food were not caused by a lack of nutritional knowledge, but that certainly made them worse. Knowing how your body reacts to things like protein and carbohydrates and then eating strategically will make your task much easier. More important, understanding nutrition for yourself and not relying on prepackaged diet food is a key to making the weight loss last.

7. Don't look to others for praise.

No amount of external praise will compensate if you feel like a failure. You can be the most organized and thoughtful soccer mom in the world and still feel empty inside. There will never be enough acclamation to cure the hurt you feel.

8. Don't buy your old excuses.

To avoid the uncomfortable task of changing our lives and getting fit, we'll tell ourselves anything. Raising small children, the demands of your job, and crowded schedules are no reason to put off your health and happiness another day. Your January 1 can come in June or any other month. And once you get started, you will be amazed at what triggers your new passions.

9. Don't wait for a sign.

It came already. You were meant to be reading this today. God is sending you signs every day—it's up to you to recognize them.

10. Recognize that this is a spiritual battle.

Nobody is meant to live an unhealthy life. This disconnect between the life we're living and the person we know we were meant to be can keep us from feeling close to God. Putting an end to that spiritual loneliness is the best reason of all to change your life.

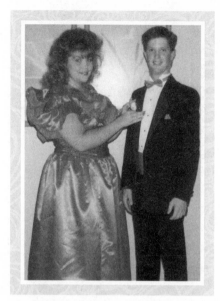

At the prom with Keith. One year after my first "successful diet," I was now bigger than before I began it!

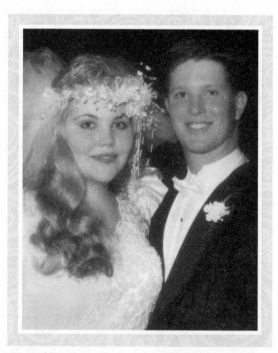

My wedding dress was a size 24. I felt like I was wearing a big white tent.

Chapter 3

Why Diets Don't Work

It's Time to Stop Being Scammed!

You might not realize it, but you are being scammed.

If you think there aren't any fat women in France, you are being scammed.

If you think bacon and eggs is the diet answer, you are being scammed.

If you think sugar is your only enemy, bust through the lie. You're being scammed.

If you think celebrities and their friend Jenny are going to help you lose weight, you are being scammed.

If you think buying that bean-shaped thing on the infomercial will make your abs look like steel, you're being scammed.

If you think L.A. has any weight-loss secrets, think again.

If you think deciding whether to spend your daily points on a slice of cheesecake or a piece of lean sirloin is the key to being slim, you may spend your entire life being scammed.

If you think football players eating lasagna and pot roast is the best system for weight loss... If you think walking for a few minutes a day is going to turn you into Jennifer Aniston...

A diet of cookies? Come on...

If you think the cobb salad is the healthy choice, you're scamming yourself.

If you have a collection of diet books that is large enough to open your own lending library, you are most definitely being scammed.

It's time to refuse the scam and let it be known that diets don't work! Temporarily, yes, but not for the long haul. A 2007 Stanford University study took 311 women, who averaged forty years old and 189 pounds, and put them on one of four diets: the low-carb Atkins and Zone diets, or the low-fat Ornish and LEARN diets. After six months the Atkins dieters had lost 13 pounds; the others, 6 to 8 pounds. But then all the dieters started to regain what they had lost. After a year the Atkins dieters had regained 3 pounds, the others 3 to 8.[1] Why the rebound? Because none of the dieters was able to stick to the plan. And even if they had, they would have trimmed only a handful of pounds.

Don't depend on a diet program to change you. You are the only one who can make the necessary decisions and then follow through to change your life. You can become as fit, toned, and healthy as you want to be. It isn't easy, but if you really want it, you will make it happen.

I know I risk offending many who believe in dieting, especially with popular diet plans. Don't forget, I spent years searching for a diet that would solve my problem too. And believe me, finding the perfect diet is not the answer. There are no magical solutions. The only permanent solution lies within you.

You can find books and programs that teach healthy lifestyle change and encourage a well-balanced diet. If you follow these programs, you will get results. And if you can stick to the program for the rest of your life, you'll experience *lasting* results. But the majority of people who wrestle with a weight problem have more fundamental struggles, and most diet programs avoid addressing this. I think I've figured out why: it's because diet programs are rigged to keep you fat. The diet industry makes more money if it can keep you on the diet teetertotter and dropping one diet in search of a new, improved program. They keep winning, and you aren't really losing.

If I had any doubts about this, they were erased in 2007 when the television show *20/20* exposed the predatory practices of one of the largest and fastest-growing weight-loss franchises. This corporation, which has centers throughout the United States, lures overweight customers with the promise of fast and affordable weight loss. There's nothing revolutionary about its program, however. The real goal is to sell clients overpriced supplements, snack bars, and protein shakes.

How does the company accomplish this? The secret is in the questionnaire you fill out during your first visit. The form includes personal questions about your past and the emotional dimension of your weight concerns. Does this weight-loss franchise pry into your personal life so its counselors can be as supportive as possible? Hardly. It's so they will have the right emotional cards to play when you come back for additional visits. They use information you supplied about yourself to break you down and convince you that weight loss is worth any price. As ex-employees revealed to *20/20*, the company's unofficial motto is "If they cry, they will buy."[2]

Watching this report made *me* want to cry. Seven years ago I was that desperate and vulnerable person who would have been summoning all my courage just to walk into a weight-loss center. I know how vulnerable people are when they begin a weight-loss program. Then the report made me mad. It's time that we break away from the diet hustlers once and for all and realize that the promises and gimmicks are designed to suck us in and sell us something. The old saying applies: if it sounds too good to be true, it probably is.

STRAIGHT TALK YOU CAN TRUST

It's time for some straight talk on diet and health. You won't like everything you're about to hear, but it will keep you from being scammed again.

Reclaiming your health and developing a lifestyle designed for fitness is not a quick fix, it doesn't rely on any secret knowledge, and it's not easy. The fitness journey you are about to embark on with me is going to be one of the hardest things you've ever done. It will require dedication, focus, and stamina. Most of all it will require belief—that you really can do this (you can!) and that God will be by your side (He will!). If this sounds like bad news to you, if you're thinking that maybe you'll give the grapefruit diet one last try, then you're not ready. If, on the other hand, you're thinking, *Bring it on!* then welcome to the club. Over time you will achieve your goal, and you'll enjoy results that last.

More on that soon. Let's take a deeper look at why the diets you and I tried in the past always failed.

Any diet plan that tells you things are going to be effortless is lying. The diet industry began with well-intentioned plans to help people lose weight. But the companies soon morphed into a sort of club that counts on lifetime members. They seek new members, of course, but it's the lifers that keep the clubs' revenues high.

This helps explain the diet-for-life clubs—the ones that have you step on a scale every week and then give you a hug no matter what the results. The good ones mean well and are giving people emotional support, which is what the companies think they need. But the underlying message is "It's okay to stay this way, as long as you show you are trying or you at least can talk about how sad you are not to be making more progress." These clubs allow people to stay in their rut by making things a little too comfortable.

I don't believe the diet industry holds secret meetings to devise new ways to sell lies. The companies simply give people what they want—a diet plan they can follow while they keep living their same old lives. No time for cardio? No problem! Work out for eight minutes in the morning, have a protein shake for lunch, and you'll lose weight! Hate vegetables? No problem! Just take the bun off your bacon cheeseburger to reduce the carbs. Better yet, if you take this pill, you won't even need food. You'll never be hungry.

> *The diet industry is giving people what they want—a diet plan they can follow while they keep living their same old lives.*

To make money for the diet industry, a program has to be attractive enough that you'll try it. The Castor Oil Diet wouldn't attract many followers. But a program that lets you eat all the meat and fat you want? Or one that lets you eat their "special" lasagna and brownies and still lose weight? Now that's worth a try!

Of course, to fly with "I want it now!" Americans, the diet also has to provide quick and impressive weight loss. If you lose 10 pounds in the first month, a couple of your friends will soon try what worked for you. By the time you discover that it's impossible to eat that way for the rest of your life, your friends have already spread the good news to their friends, even as their own diet attempts start to break down.

In this way a diet program is like a virus—you get it, spread it, and then get over it while others continue to catch it. Like those who followed the four diet plans in the Stanford University study, people lose a little weight for the first few months. Somewhere around six months, they start to rebound, but by then everyone has heard how so-and-so lost 15 pounds on the ____ Diet. That's why new diet plans can have phenomenal success for a couple of years, until everybody compares notes and says, "You know? When all was said and done, we didn't lose any weight!"

The truth is that many of the leading diets provide excellent basic advice—and I'll go over all that in part 2 of this book. But few diets ask you to do the hard inner work that's necessary *before* you begin watching calories and lacing up your sneakers.

YOU CAN CHANGE—FOR GOOD

For the majority of people, diets fail if they make us feel like we're not in control. I resent being told what to do. Plus, when we are simply following orders, we never take personal responsibility. We are foot soldiers with no say in what happens to us. What I discovered about myself is that I needed to be the general of my weight-loss battle. I understand that some personality types thrive on positive reinforcement—whether they achieve their fitness goals or not. But for me, the last thing I needed was ritualistic comfort. Accountability, yes, but too much unconditional support would have derailed me. My desire to change was powered by how *uncomfortable* I was in my own skin. I didn't want anyone trying to make me feel good about staying the way I was.

I wanted to change because I was tired of how other people reacted to me and because I wanted to live a normal life, shop in normal stores, sit in normal seats. But more than that, I wanted to accomplish something great. I didn't want to have surgery that would cause me to lose weight only because a doctor rerigged my digestive system. I wanted to take responsibility for myself and lose weight, proving that I could do it. I also feared I'd gain back the weight if I had surgery, because I'd never learn self-control if the control was taken away.

As bad as the diet scammers are, the new generation of diet scientists may be even worse. They tell the public that permanent weight loss is virtually impossible. They've done the studies and found that 98 percent of those who lose weight gain it all back. They say they believe the body has a preset natural weight and while you might be able to change it by 10 or 20 pounds, you can't do more than that. These scientists follow in the tradition of the people who said the four-minute mile couldn't be broken, a woman could never swim the English Channel, and a man could never come back from three types of cancer to win seven Tours de France. They study what *most* people do and seem to forget that exceptional performances happen all the time when people put their minds to a task and persevere.

If the rule is that everyone who loses weight gains it back, then I am an exception to the rule. So are thousands of others who have lost weight and kept it off for years. In so doing, we've reclaimed our lives. We've rediscovered our joy and passion. The diet police would do well to stop studying the people who rebound at six months and start paying attention to those of us who get fit, stay that way, and know there's no going back.

This book will help you become one of the exceptional success stories. You don't need to be superhuman to make it happen. You just need to ignore the naysayers, keep your eyes on the prize, and go for it with all your heart and soul. It worked for me, and it can work for you too.

Promise yourself that you'll never be scammed again. Make up your mind to own your issues and look them dead on. My passion is for giving hope and proving that exceptional things happen—despite conventional wisdom. You and I are people, not statistics. We can beat the odds and get lasting results.

THE LIMITS OF DIETING

Ever wonder why so many weight-loss books present a trendy new diet plan but very few focus on the exercise side of the fitness equation? Because it's hard to make money by telling people the simple truth: go work out for an hour each day, and you'll lose weight!

Controlling food intake is an important part of weight management, but to lose weight you still need to burn more calories than you take in. That's why exercise is crucial. When you cut back drastically on your daily food intake, at first you'll lose weight. But your body is very sophisticated, and once it senses that less food might be a regular thing, it starts adjusting. It slows your metabolism down so you burn fewer calories throughout the day. It depresses your system—and that can be depressing! You get sluggish. You have little energy. You act less like a bird and more like a turtle on a cold day. And you stop losing weight.

That is a big problem with all diets, and it explains why studies are documenting the six-month rebound. People lose weight at first, but once their bodies adjust to lower calorie intake, the weight loss stops. Worse, they now have slowed metabolisms, so if they fall off the diet and return to their old eating habits, they regain all their weight and more!

To lose weight, I knew I had to hold myself to a sane number of calories per day. More important, I had to concentrate on the activity side of the weight-loss equation. Cardiovascular activity keeps your metabolism high, not just during exercise but for hours afterward. And more muscle also raises your metabolism. I know I promised to keep the math to a minimum in this book, but here's one number you'll want to know: it takes nine times as much energy to turn food into muscle as it does to turn food into fat. Every pound of muscle you add means 9 pounds of fat you're *not* adding.

To get fit, you need to eat right, and you need to exercise. It's not one or the other; it's both.

—•••••—

From the Mouths of Babes

When my son Luke was three years old, he came home from preschool with a Mother's Day gift. It was a letter that his teacher had filled in for him, describing things about his mommy. Here's what Luke's sheet said:

When I'm at school, she is...working out at the gym.

For fun, she likes to...run.

Her favorite food is...celery, salad, and carrots.

She likes to have me help her...make helfy snacks.

I love her because she...takes care of me.

I had to laugh, because I remembered my older daughter, Ashley, filling out the same card years earlier, long before I made the decisions that changed my life. Here's Ashley's list:

When I'm at school, she is...watching *Regis and Kathie Lee*

For fun, she likes to...bake cakes

Her favorite food is...cakes

She likes to have me help her...make cookies

I love her because she...makes good food

When I compare the two lists and think about the changes that have taken place, it's hilarious and sad and great, all at the same time. My kids and your kids learn from what we do far more than from what we say. So start living in a new way. It will transform your health, and it will be a daily lesson in healthy living for your children. Every day is the right day to be the best you can be!

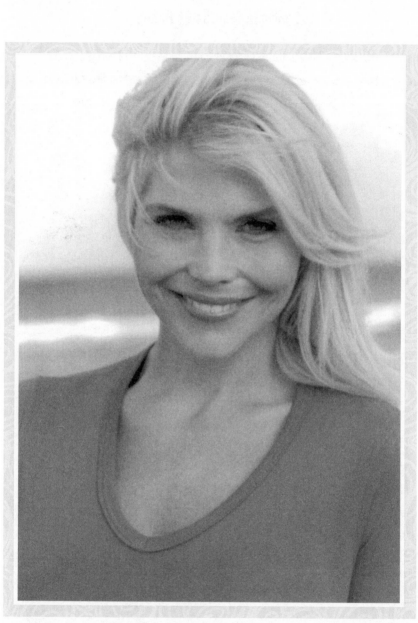

It's still awesome some days to remind myself that I don't ever have to go back. I get to be the new me for the rest of my life!

Chapter 4

No Looking Back

Is This Your Turning Point?

Believe it or not, the second half of my journey has delivered more emotional triumph than the first half had pain. The morning of April 30, 2001, I opened my eyes and realized my life was beginning all over again. It was both exciting and terrifying. Exciting, because I was finally going to become the person I was meant to be. Terrifying, because I had no idea how I was going to do it.

But I did know there was no looking back. I also knew:

1. I had made a deal with God the night before. That was nonnegotiable.

2. I had declared my intentions to my husband. If I quit, he'd know it. He wouldn't say anything about it, but if I failed, it would be a constant reminder that I had broken a promise.

3. I needed to learn more about nutrition, but I wasn't interested in a diet plan. I'd tried enough of those to know they didn't work for me. I needed to do something that would play to my strengths and negate my weaknesses.

4. I needed to set goals—big ones and small ones—so I'd always have a way to measure my success.

5. Achieving my weight-loss goal was going to take a long time. But that was okay, because the new me was something I'd be for the rest of my life. I had a brand-new outlook.

6. My body needed to *move!*

7. I was sick of failure. I was desperate to be proud of myself, not just to put on a "pretty face." During the first several months, anytime I started to waver in my plan, I reminded myself how miserable it would feel to fail again and how desperate my cry to God had been. Any amount of self-sacrifice was better than going back to the way I was before.

8. The greatest realization was this: God would be with me every step of the way. He never quits, and He never loses. If I ever felt like I didn't have the strength to continue, I would always find strength in God. He held all the power for me to succeed in my new life, and He would give it to me every time I asked.

When I thought about my previous dieting attempts, I realized that none of the plans I'd tried had failed me. *I had failed the plans.* Any of the leading diet plans could have taken off a few pounds if I had eaten exactly as they told me and exercised regularly. But I hadn't been able to stick with them. I would fall off the wagon after realizing I couldn't eat the way the plan required for the rest of my life.

And it wasn't just me. I knew plenty of people who had stopped and started over every Monday, just like I did. It was as if we were pretending to be dieters, but eventually we couldn't stay in character any longer.

I had to change my fundamental relationship with food and exercise. I had to change my mind-set so my brain would eventually seek healthy, low-calorie food and vigorous activity.

But how to do it?

Answer: One step at a time. One day at a time. One success at a time.

First, Change Your Mind

As I thought about how to begin, I decided not to mess with my eating habits during the first month. This was a marathon, not a sprint. My number one priority was not to fail; I didn't want to jeopardize that by tackling too much at once. As long as I kept making progress, the speed of my progress was not so important.

Establishing an exercise habit was goal number one, and I knew it wouldn't be easy. Like many overweight people, I hated exercise. I'd accompanied my husband to the gym a few times in halfhearted efforts to make myself feel better whenever the self-hatred got particularly intense. But the combination of physical discomfort, perceived public humiliation, and pathetic performance was about as much fun as a root canal. Actually, I'd have chosen the root canal.

But, like it or not, that had to change. One, I was going to have to live with the discomfort. Fine. I was ready to choose physical pain over the pain of desperation. Two, there were going to be some embarrassing moments. Fine again. To accomplish anything that's important, you have to set aside your pride. And what was my pride getting me, anyway? Three, my pathetic performance didn't matter. The only person I'd be measuring myself against would be me. As long as I kept improving and showing up, I'd be right on track.

I chose to exercise that first day at a gym. I was anxious to get going, and

I already had a membership, so I put on sweats and a big T-shirt and headed out. The gym had recumbent bikes—the ones where you sit in a more chair-like position—which I figured was my best bet. I could sit and not worry about people watching my shape from behind. Walking or running was completely out of the question. I could last only a few minutes, and I had committed to exercise for thirty minutes with intensity.

I walked in the gym, smiled at Dan, the front-desk guy, and hopped on the first bike I came to. I didn't want to go any farther into the gym than I had to. And I wanted to be close to the door so I could get out as soon as I hit thirty minutes.

I began pedaling. Almost immediately I started breathing hard, but that was okay. I just slowed down a little and kept going. I kept the resistance level at five—pretty easy. I pushed myself as much as possible but not so much that I'd collapse. My goal was to go for thirty minutes without stopping, no matter what. And I made it! I stepped off that bike sore and sweat soaked but having tasted clean success for the first time in memory. What a sweet feeling!

Since my goal was to establish a new exercise habit, I needed consistency, consistency, consistency. No debating *whether* I wanted to exercise every day. I treated it as my new job. I had to show up six days a week, no matter how I felt or how I might be influenced by outside circumstances. As with starting any new job, I figured I had no vacation or sick time coming. I did let myself take Sundays off. If I didn't give myself one break day a week, it would start to feel more like prison than a job.

Every day that first week I walked into the gym, said hi to Dan, and hopped on my bike. I have to hand it to Dan. He always made me feel like he was happy to see me. If the gym had had a condescending greeter, I still would have stuck to my plan (remember, there are *no excuses*), but he made it easy to show up. There was childcare at the gym too, which made things convenient. And sometimes I would sneak off to the gym first thing in the morning, while Keith and the kids were still sleeping.

That first week I stayed at level five on the bike's resistance. The next week I went up to level ten. I quickly understood what they meant by "feel the burn." Then I started pushing myself to level fifteen for short bursts, and by the end of the first month, I was pedaling up to level fifteen every session. I can't express how incredible it felt to experience something other than disappointment. This was cool! That's why my exercise program wasn't that hard once I got started. Of course it was physically and mentally draining, and there were days I'd have to drag myself to the gym, but once I drove off the parking lot after exercising, I instantly felt so much better about myself and my future.

Having clear measures of my progress was exactly what I needed. That's another plus of a stationary bike. On the readout you can see how many calories you're burning, what level you're working at, and how fast you're pedaling. I could see that I was getting better every day. I could make a game of it. This was now Mission: Possible. I needed the encouragement of seeing I was making progress; if my only measure had been weighing myself, I'd have been disappointed. It takes some time before your work efforts show up as significant weight loss. And I knew better than to rely on the compliments of other people. When you are severely overweight, you need to lose a lot before people even notice.

By the end of that first month, however, I had lost a few pounds. More important, I had met my first goal. One day Dan said, "Wow, you've been here every day!"

I smiled. "And I will be here tomorrow and the day after that."

EXERCISE ALONE WON'T DO IT

I was ready to set a big goal, and I knew just what it should be. My thirtieth birthday was eight months away. Would it be possible to lose 100 pounds by then? What could be a better symbol of my commitment to a new life than celebrating the beginning of a new decade as a healthy and fit person? I decided to go for it. It would happen.

But I had to confront my eating habits. No way was I gonna make it if I kept dancing with the glazed croissants. I needed a self-taught course in nutrition, but in the meantime I resolved to simply eat less. I wasn't ready to give up my favorite foods, because I knew from experience that trying to eat stuff you hate leads to failure. I once tried a diet that required cottage cheese every day. Cottage cheese is disgusting. I held my nose for three days but couldn't do it after that. End of another diet.

I stuck with my favorites—it was still fettuccine alfredo for dinner—but I made a conscious effort to stop a few bites short of what I wanted. I would even put a portion on a small salad plate so it seemed like more and limit myself to that. I tried to always walk away from the table slightly hungry. It was very, very difficult. Your body's natural instinct is definitely not to walk away from food while you're still hungry! But I made some modest improvements. Even if it didn't make a huge caloric difference, I was learning self-control. And that was a whole new concept for me.

Then, as I kept improving on the recumbent bike, I introduced myself to the world of nutrition. I read everything I could get my hands on. I learned what a carbohydrate is. I also checked out the Atkins diet, which everyone I knew was doing, but it didn't appeal to me. Sausage and steak have never been my things.

I learned about the principles of hibernation; that stuck with me. A body can burn either carbohydrates or fats for fuel. But carbohydrates are a lot easier to burn, so given the choice, your body will use the carbs you're feeding it and leave the fat on your thighs in case you find yourself in a famine. Only when your body runs out of carbs will it start liquidating its fat supplies. That's what happens with hibernating creatures—while they sleep through the winter, they slowly burn stored fat. I needed to keep my carbs to a minimum so I could start burning my fat.

I also needed to eat smaller, more frequent meals to keep my metabolism high and to prevent powerful hunger attacks from triggering a binge response. I learned that a hefty dinner is particularly deadly, because that late in the day your body has no way to burn off the calories. As your activity decreases at bedtime, the extra calories get stored as fat.

I decided to eat five meals a day of about 300 calories each. I had a protein shake for breakfast, then some fruit and plain lunchmeat as a midmorning snack. For the next six months, I had the same sandwich for lunch *every day*. I can recite the ingredients in my sleep: two slices of honey-baked turkey, a sandwich-stacker pickle, about half a head of lettuce, a slice of onion, wholegrain bread, and just enough mayo to make the turkey stick to the bread.

No doubt that sounds incredibly boring—maybe even depressing—to you. But that's the point. I *needed* food to be boring. Food had been my major source of entertainment for twenty-nine years, and it had practically ruined my life! We will talk a lot about this later in the book. For now, just understand that I had to break the power that food held over my life. I needed to start thinking of food as fuel, not fun. Eating the same sandwich every day wasn't depressing at all. It gave me great pleasure to eat with discipline.

Eating around 1,500 calories a day left me a little hungry but never ravenous. That, I learned, is key. Being mildly hungry is not such a bad feeling, especially when you remind yourself that mild hunger is what it feels like for your body to burn fat. Being ravenous, on the other hand, is unworkable. Diets that leave you starving throughout much of the day are going to backfire. By having a small meal every few hours, I kept myself from ever losing control. And I knew I didn't need to feel full, because it wouldn't be long before I'd be eating again.

My midafternoon snack might be a protein bar or some popcorn and fruit. Dinner would be grilled chicken and some salad or other veggies. Natural, wholesome, low carb, and high protein. It was, and is, a smart way to eat.

As far as beverages go, I tried to make sure I didn't drink my calories. I've read that the average American drinks more than 300 calories a day. Juice and alcohol are as loaded with calories as soda is. I stuck to water and zero-cal diet drinks.

Being mildly hungry is not such a bad feeling. It's what it feels like for your body to burn fat.

That month I also tried a treadmill for the first time. I was getting pretty good on the bike, so how hard could a treadmill be? Well, thirty minutes on a treadmill at a somewhat snail-like pace of three miles per hour had my heart rate so rapid that I felt like I was going to be sick. If you had told me that one day I'd run ten miles on a treadmill, I'd have said you were full of it. I did walk on a treadmill, which I couldn't have done a month earlier. I stuck to it and kept moving faster.

After a few months of exercise, I decided to tackle the elliptical trainer. It was such a popular machine that I thought it must work magic. My best friend, Judi, could do sixty minutes on the elliptical, and she was my hero. My first time, as my feet glided back and forth at 300-plus pounds, I couldn't stay on a full two minutes. It was intense. A few days later my goal was five minutes. I barely made it, sweat pouring, barely breathing. My next goal was ten minutes, then fifteen. A couple of months later I could do my whole thirty minutes on the elliptical. Again, I was competing with myself and winning. A huge personal accomplishment! And another goal checked off.

HOW TO KEEP FROM GIVING UP

What you want to know is, was I tempted to stop? Of course I was! Every day. Every time I didn't want to work out or wanted to eat an ice-cream sundae with my kids, I had to remind myself how miserable I was being fat. Escaping misery is a powerful motivator. I would say to myself, "Chantel, how unhappy are you fat? If you cheat now, you've gotta stay fat another day." Even after I could afford to cheat occasionally, I was so ready to have that monkey off my back.

I was replacing an old source of pleasure with one that fit my new life. The pleasure of celebrating milestones was taking the place once reserved for food. The endorphins from the exercise itself felt great—and stayed with me for hours—and knowing that I was accomplishing something really hard and worthwhile felt even better. Few pleasures in life can compete with dropping your big old clothes at Goodwill and buying new, smaller outfits.

The upshot? I did it! By January 30, 2002, I had lost 101 pounds. Never in my life had I achieved anything like that. And my husband and I threw the biggest party of our lives. Keith planned it, and we invited more than one hundred people—all my best friends, of course, but also many people whom I hadn't seen in a year. It was my coming-out party, so of course I needed a really special outfit. I looked and looked and looked. Finally at Macy's I found a gorgeous pair of size 14 beaded black pants—in the ladies department! For the first time since I was a kid, I didn't have to shop in the plus-size department, hidden in a distant corner.

The party was unforgettable. I mingled and chatted and danced all night. And unlike my sweet-sixteen birthday party, this time I got to enjoy a piece of my own cake.

A few things stand out in my mind from that night. One was a friend's husband who said, "Wow, Chantel, you've lost a lot of weight!"

"Thanks," I said.

"That's great. But it doesn't matter," he continued. "You'll probably gain it all back."

"What?"

"Everybody does. I've lost and regained 50 pounds more times than I can tell you."

I couldn't believe it. Here I'd lost 100 pounds, I was celebrating my new life, I was on a roll, and this goofball rained on my parade. Of course, he was just one of many people over the years who have told me that I'd probably go back to being my old self. They didn't understand that for me it was about so much more than weight loss. I had made the Five Decisions that changed the way I thought about myself, my life, my health, and my future. I had undergone a Brain Change, a new way of thinking that directed me into a new way of living. I now had a new "normal"; I would never go back to being the same.

My greatest memories from that party are of a couple of photos. One is a shot of Keith and me, and there are two things sticking out from my neck. Collarbones! I had collarbones! Who knew?

The other photo is of seven close girlfriends and me, all lined up and turned toward the camera at the same angle, like a chorus line. When I saw the picture, I was blown away. In every photo that had been taken of me, I felt I stood out like an elephant in a herd of giraffes. But the eight of us were lined up, and I totally blended in. I was now one of the girls.

Strength Training and a Call from *Oprah*

During the next year I worked out harder than ever. I took up Spinning and began strength training. I had learned that strength training—lifting weights or any exercise that gives muscles intense resistance—is the best way to build a lean body. It doesn't necessarily burn as many calories as cardiovascular exercise while you're doing it, but it does a lot more to tone your body. And by building muscle, you raise your metabolism. Because muscle burns more energy than fat does, I constantly remind my clients that cardio burns calories for today, while strength training burns them for tomorrow. Both are vital for a complete exercise program.

I can't say enough about how strength training transformed my body. For example, I was asked to be a bridesmaid at a family wedding. I went to be measured and was told by the saleswoman to order a size 14 dress. Well, I didn't like the sound of that, so I had her order a size 10. She resisted; I insisted. A few months later when the dress finally arrived, it had to be *taken in*.

But you know what? The actual weight loss was starting to slow down. I dropped 65 pounds over the next eight months—fantastic by any normal standards but sometimes frustrating for me. Crazy, huh? I had become so obsessed with losing 2 to 3 pounds a week that anything less felt like failure. I had to consciously tell myself that I wasn't slacking off, that I was still giving it my all.

In any case, I was nearly there. Down to about 165 pounds. Getting fit. I could see light at the end of the tunnel. But I was about to face the biggest test of my journey so far.

We had just returned from a family vacation in the mountains of North Carolina, and things were going great. I ran in the mountains. I even took some resistance bands—and used them. Coming home in the car, I started to feel a subtle nausea creep over me, an unmistakable sensation. By that point in my life, I knew it well.

Was I pregnant? Six tests later, every one with two lines, I knew I was.

On one hand I was overjoyed. A new baby! On the other I was terrified. For two years my life had been focused on watching the scale go down. That was the measure of my success. How long would it take me just to get back to where I was that day? What if I *never* got back? And how would I find time for exercise with *four* children?

No matter what happened, I'd promised myself and God that I would be the best I could be. Being pregnant would last for the next nine months, but being the best pregnant woman didn't mean a big bowl of ice cream every night. My mission was still the same. The journey continued.

Before I even started to show, I got an exciting phone call. An *Oprah Winfrey Show* producer said they wanted me to appear on an "Incredible Weight-Loss Stories" episode. I almost fell over. I had sent the show my before-and-after photos just five days earlier. Now they wanted me in Chicago—the very next week! I was going to meet Oprah! This was exactly the new focus I needed. Not only would I get a chance to show the world how hard I'd worked and what I'd done, but I could inspire other women who didn't think it was possible. That was what God had wanted from me. And now it was really happening.

I went on the show four-months pregnant, but no one could tell. The experience was like a fairy tale. I stood backstage watching a monitor as Oprah introduced me. On the screen a montage of videos and still photos from my past played as my voice told the story of my struggle. It dawned on me that sixty-five million people were watching my body dancing around at 340 pounds. Before that could sink in, the cameras panned the audience. Keith was sobbing. My mom and my friends who had accompanied me were all sobbing too. I started to cry a few tears but managed to hold it together as Oprah called me on stage. It was surreal to be sitting up there. Here was this woman I admired tremendously. I had so many questions I'd have loved to ask her, but instead we were talking about me. Ironic. Things went smoothly, and the audience seemed to really respond. I left Chicago praying that someone somewhere now believed a new life was possible.

The coolest part of the experience came at the end of the taping. One of the producers had asked me before I came to Chicago to name one thing I regretted about being fat. There were so many, but whenever I looked at my wedding pictures, it always irritated me that I had let myself be a fat bride. I'd missed out on having wedding pictures that I could show with pride.

Backstage, the stylist had pulled together an entire room of stunning wedding dresses for me to choose from and had told me not to breathe a word of this to Keith. At the end of the show, I came out on stage in a new wedding dress, carrying a bouquet of roses, and got to pull Keith on stage with me. It was a magical moment. I was given the dress as a gift, and a few weeks later we renewed our marriage vows on our tenth anniversary. I felt like a bride again—and had an album full of pictures to be proud of.

After the whirlwind of *Oprah,* it took a little time to readjust to my ordinary life. Soon I was starting to show. Many days I would get on the scale and watch it go up a pound or two, and I would start to cry. "I'm never going to get back to where I was!"

Finally Keith hid the scale. He grabbed my shoulders and looked straight at me. "Honey, you're pregnant!" he said. "You're eating well. You're exercising. It's nothing you can change. It's the way it has to work; we want a healthy baby!"

For a while I wanted my scale back, but eventually I let it go. Then I started to feel a little better. Without the scale close, I could let my brain keep me on track. Weight was not the issue as much as keeping my commitment to healthy living.

In June 2003, Luke was born. The tears I'd cried upon finding out I was pregnant seemed unimaginable when I held this perfect baby in my arms. Yet, a few weeks later I fell into a classic postpartum depression. I didn't feel like a fitness phenomenon. I had to get back to serious work, only now I was a sleep-deprived mom with four kids. But I went back on my eating plan and made myself start exercising again as soon as the doctor approved it. Normal life returned.

FACING A FAMILY CRISIS

Two months later I received a terrible phone call from my dad. After eleven years of excellent health, my mom was sick again with leukemia. I nearly lost it. How could God let this happen? Why now? Would my mom survive this time? And how could I juggle my exercise and my family and be a source of strength to her?

I was home folding clothes with the television on. A familiar gospel song began to play, with words about taking things a day at a time. In that instant I knew I had my answer. I had to trust God and keep moving forward one day at a time. I immediately called my mom in the hospital, sang the song to her, and reassured her we would be okay.

How important was my mission if it couldn't survive a family illness or the birth of a child? There is no valid reason to stop taking care of yourself, just opportunities for excuses. And if excuses are what you're looking for, they will show up. I'd been occasionally tempted to use a crisis or unexpected development to give up on my new life. But with prayer I managed to turn away, always remembering my old pain.

At the same time, I redoubled my fitness efforts. We all find time for the things we care about most. For me, that involved begging my husband to do diaper duty for thirty minutes so I could go to the gym (and then taking an hour!), running with a Baby Jogger, and doing my strength training at home while Luke napped. It involved cutting back on things like television and, yes, sometimes sleep.

Many days I had to read and reread one of my favorite passages from the Bible: "Consider it pure joy, my brothers, whenever you face trials of many kinds, because you know that the testing of your faith develops perseverance" (James 1:2–3). Perseverance and I had become best friends. These trials would make me better. God promised it. And over time, my depression was defeated.

Four months after having Luke I had lost all of my pregnancy weight and the other 10 pounds I wanted to lose. Best of all, my mom was in remission!

LIVING A NEW LIFE

At some point my journey stopped being about weight loss. Staying active now comes automatically to me, as it will for you once you've carved that habit into your brain. And although I no longer focus on weight, I feel like I'm still on the same journey that started years ago when I reached a point of desperation. From the beginning my goal has been to become the best person I can be. It's a daily quest that has taken a lot of different twists and turns, some I never could have expected.

What has changed is that I no longer need to accomplish goals for the purpose of getting praise from others. All I need is God's approval. The scars of my previous low self-esteem continue to fade a little more all the time. I know that probably a hint will always remain. That's fine, because to me those scars are a beautiful reminder. They give me a story to tell of hope and of God's faithfulness. I am the person I am today because of who I once was.

• • • • • •

Ten Things to Expect—Some Good, and Some Even Better

1. **It's not primarily about looking good.**

   For me, walking around fat was like wearing a T-shirt that said "I'm worthless—please like me anyway." Losing weight was my way of taking control of my life and of changing my relationships with others. Every time I was tempted to quit, I had to remind myself how miserable I had been when I was fat. If changing my life had just been about vanity, I might not have made the changes permanent.

2. **Set goals.**

   It's not a journey unless you have a destination. You need to envision the person you want to be, and right away you need to start thinking like that person. On the other hand, don't feel like you need to achieve your goal in a week. Are you bettering yourself every day? Great! That's what matters.

3. **Don't set yourself up for failure.**

   God made you to move. It's a basic pleasure in life but one that you may need to rediscover. If you're like me, you are convinced that you'll hate exercise, but that won't last. Finding an activity you love and a comfortable environment for doing it is fundamental to your success. I didn't deal with my food issues at all until I'd established an exercise habit. And I didn't try any intense workouts until I got comfortable with the recumbent bike. Becoming a whole different person is not easy, so take baby steps.

4. Great accomplishments require great sacrifice.

When was the last time you took the trash out and felt great about the accomplishment? To feel incredibly proud of yourself, you must pick some hard tasks and put your all into achieving them. Nothing worthwhile is easy.

5. It's not the diet; it's you!

If you follow some of the leading diet and exercise plans and do exactly what they prescribe, you'll lose weight. The problem with these diets is that they have little understanding of the human brain and an individual's ingrained food obsessions. Until you've changed your brain and reset your internal drives, no diet plan will deliver lasting results.

6. You will be hungry.

Most overweight people have gotten used to consuming serious calories on a daily basis without even realizing it. When you reduce your caloric intake, at first your body will scream for more. It doesn't need the calories, but it *thinks* it does. And that's all hunger is—your body sending you a signal that it wants more. It doesn't necessarily mean you *need* more.

There's no getting around this, and it doesn't feel good. Any diet plan that says you won't get hungry is lying. But as long as you keep eating small and more frequent meals, the hunger will be manageable. When the signal gets strong and you learn to ignore it, you're developing the skill of self-control, which you'll use in all sorts of ways to achieve success in life.

7. Educating yourself is essential.

Understanding the ways different foods affect your health and hunger and ways you'll benefit from various exercises is essential for personalizing your Brain-Change plan. The chapters in part 2 of this book will get you started. The diet industry treats you like you can't think for yourself, which is why so many require you to use their prepackaged food. I'll let you in on a secret: if you buy in to their plan, you will need to buy their food for the rest of your life. But if you learn to develop a new, healthy relationship with food, you will ensure permanent change. And *you* will be in control.

8. *You don't have to be Wonder Woman.*

I'm no superhero. I'm just an ordinary wife and mother. I take care of my kids. I cook meals. I drive my kids to cheerleading practice and T-ball games. I go shopping with my friends. I don't come from a long line of ultra-athletes. The life I've re-created for myself has come from determination and making daily decisions about what I eat and how I spend my time. I am just like you. You don't have to be Wonder Woman; you just have to want it enough to make it happen.

9. *Count on disappointments, obstacles, setbacks, and life crises.*

Over the course of my fitness journey, I've dealt with unexpected pregnancy, postpartum depression, job losses, a serious auto accident, sick parents, the deaths of loved ones, and many other rough patches. I've had many opportunities to cut back on my workouts so I'd have more time to deal with a crisis, or to binge on sweets because I was emotionally spent. But there is no real excuse to go off course. Once you have chosen this path, you are on it for good. Adversity is the glue that makes you stronger!

10. *Take time to celebrate.*

Even if a producer from *Oprah* doesn't call this week, you need to schedule regular events to remind yourself how far you've come. Birthday parties, special dinners, a new outfit in a smaller size—rewards sweeten the sacrifice. Don't cheat yourself out of the joy that comes with creating a new life.

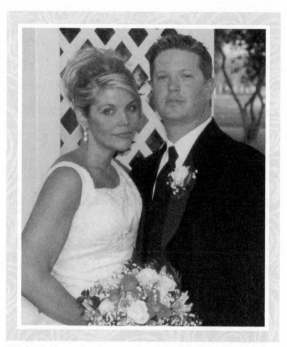

With Keith on the day we renewed our vows. I'm wearing the wedding dress I received as a gift when I appeared on Oprah.

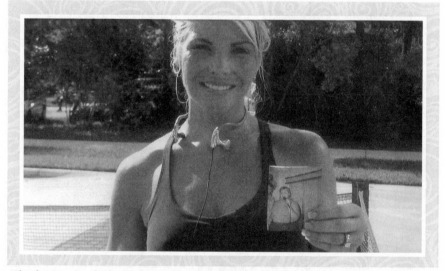

The day I realized I had left the miserable woman behind. This was taken in 2004 after my first race. I'm holding a photo that I carried the entire time to remind myself of how far I had come and that I could finish strong.

Chapter 5

When Was Your Last Peak Moment?

It's Time to Take Your Life Off Pause

I remember every detail of the time I fell in love with exercise. It was 2002, and I walked into my first Spinning class. I had been on my weight-loss journey for about six months. I was eating right and was using a recumbent bike, but I wasn't loving it. I was down from 349 pounds to 262, but I was still a big girl, and the moment I walked into that Spinning class, I was completely intimidated.

Spinning is like using a stationary bike but on a whole different level. The bike's pedals are connected to the flywheel, so even if you stop pedaling, the pedals—and your feet—keep moving. You can't really stop. More important, Spinning incorporates interval training, climbing with resistance, jogging in a standing position, motivational instruction, powerful music, and visualization exercises to turn indoor biking into a superintense and invigorating experience. Lance Armstrong could train for the Tour on a Spinner.

When I walked into my first Spinning class, I wondered what I was in for—and soon found out. Everyone climbed on their bikes to loosen up. The twelve bikes were arranged in a semicircle facing the instructor, with a wall mirror behind her. With that mirror staring me down, it was impossible to ignore the fact that I was twice the size of anyone else in the class. Was I self-conscious? Oh yeah! But I was ready to lay down a little pride. I started pedaling.

The other thing that couldn't be ignored was how much that tiny, hard seat hurt my 260-pound frame. You'd think my extra cushioning would have helped, but not with that bicycle seat. After about one minute I started to feel winded and decided to step off the bike and save my energy. Class hadn't even started yet!

When class did start, I climbed back on, and away we went. Within five minutes I was spent. Meanwhile, the two senior citizens in the class weren't even breathing hard. Then the instructor told us to stand up and pedal for five minutes, as if we were climbing a hill. I thought, *What kind of sick joke is this?* Everyone began the trek to the top, but within a minute I was ready to head back down. That's one great thing about Spinning—the instructor encourages you to push your limits, but you decide when enough is enough, and you control how much resistance there is on your Spinner. That first day I had to pace myself carefully, and I stayed seated throughout most of the forty-five-minute class, but I finished! For me, it was a phenomenal peak moment! They would have had to haul me out of there on a stretcher before I would have quit.

At the end of the session, I dragged myself off the bike, totally drained. I didn't look like I'd been in combat; I looked like I'd *died* in combat! I'd never been so exhausted, but I was also bursting with pride! It was strange, but I immediately felt strong. I ran to my car, called one of my best friends, and screamed, "You're never going to believe it. I did my first Spinning class!" I had a sense that anything that hard had the potential to make me really, really fit. I was right.

That first Spinning experience was painful, daunting, and even a bit scary, but powerful. I was hooked! The next morning when I woke up aching all over, all I could think about was how to drag my butt out of bed so I could take another class. And I did, that day. And I've been going back ever since.

Spinning made me realize something. For too many years I hadn't looked forward to anything. I hadn't had enough peak moments—those times when you accomplish something important to you. When you experience a peak moment, all the fluff of life gets burned away, and you suddenly see yourself, your life, and your purpose with clarity. You feel you are making your life happen as it should.

For most of us, those moments are few and far between. For me, the only ones I remembered from my earlier life were my high-school graduation, my wedding day, and the births of my children. There had been thousands of unmemorable days in between and a few I wished to forget. But after that night driving alone in the car, when I was so desperate I knew I *had* to change, something began to shift. And after that first Spinning class, when I was so excited that I had to tell a friend all about it, something definitely shifted. Whatever had been clogging the gears of my life came loose, and everything began to move faster and smoother and better. Since that day I have peak moments *all the time.* Don't buy the lie that peak moments should be rare, sprinkled through your life ever so sparingly. They should be the meat of life! If I haven't tasted a satisfying peak moment in a few weeks, I know something is off, and I do what I need to get back on track.

When Was Your Last Peak Moment?

Most of us let other people or life circumstances dictate our peak moments. It's easy to fall into the habit of waiting for a performance review at work or compliments on our home or our appearance to affirm our accomplishments. It's great to accept the praise of others, of course, but don't restrict your peak moments to the times other people notice you're doing a fabulous job.

Let your peak moments begin within you. Set regular goals, and feel the glow of achievement when you reach them. Every day I wake up looking forward to working toward the next goal. It's a big change from when I used to wake up looking forward to cookies.

You could say that I traded the pleasure of sugar for the pleasure of peak moments, which is a far more exciting way to live. I firmly believe that if I could take every person in America who has a food issue and let them experience a genuine peak moment—an earned achievement—most of those food issues would disappear. People would realize what they are *really* after, and it isn't made by Ben and Jerry.

So I ask you: when was your last peak moment? If you can't remember, that's a sure sign you need to change the way you think about your life. Stop settling for the momentary pleasures of food, television, and long naps on the couch. A higher level of joy and fulfillment is waiting for you! Refuse to settle for a mediocre life.

Unfit people often want to improve their health and looks but dread the "torture" of exercise. I encounter that attitude all the time, and it's completely backward. Start working out because it feels great. Then enjoy the side effects: improved health and a fit body.

I'm not saying that exercise isn't hard. It is, if you're pushing your limits and staying committed. What I'm saying is that hard work is underrated. We've come to believe that the ultimate life involves the luxury of gadgets and hired help to take care of everything for us so we never have to break a sweat. That's a lie! You are blessed to be alive, and not being active shows a lack of gratitude for the gift of life. Don't waste precious time sitting on the couch. You exist in a physical body, and you are meant to use that body. What are you saving it for?

We prevent ourselves from excelling by overmothering ourselves. When you constantly check in with yourself—*Am I exhausted? Am I hungry? Am I cold? Am I tired? How do I feel today?*—you don't achieve personal bests. Instead, you're nurturing self-centeredness. But when you stop thinking and start doing, you go further than you thought you could. And you feel really, really strong.

Spinning is not the only fitness program that has figured out ways to help people achieve this, but it gave me what I needed. When you are in the middle of that group of bikers and you feel like the group is racing down the Alps in the Tour de France, it's quite a rush! You feel powerful, like you can do anything. If you are one of those people who always thought of exercise as something that was good for you but unpleasant, like going to the dentist, then you are in for a wonderful surprise.

Get Ready to Change Your Life

One day during the week of my thirtieth birthday, our Spinning instructor failed to show up, so I volunteered to teach the class. It was the coolest thing I ever did. I realized how far I'd come from my first time on a recumbent bike. Another peak moment! I, Chantel Hobbs, former fat girl, was teaching a Spinning class. My family couldn't believe it. I decided then and there to become an instructor.

After I got certified, I started teaching at my gym. I was very comfortable there. Everyone knew me, loved my story, and loved seeing me transform my life. Soon after, I was asked to start teaching at another gym too, three times a week. Panic attack! I was pretty fit, but I had more weight to lose. I was still over 200 pounds. Yet I was not about to let the opportunity go. I was so gung-ho about teaching that I'd have taught in the middle of the night if they'd wanted me to. But I was nervous. I didn't look like the typical instructor. I thought, *These people are going to think, "Oh, so this is what Spinning does for you—great!"*

Did I act nervous for that first class? No way! I walked in like I owned the room. Everyone was wonderful, and I had a blast. I ended up teaching there for three years. I still remember the first time my mother took one of my classes. She sobbed through the whole thing. She said she never thought she'd see the day. I felt so proud, showing her that I had become a person who inspires others.

Spinning changed the way I approach life. In fact, it's an incredible metaphor. It's like you're climbing the mountain of life, pedal by pedal. When I tell people we're going to climb for twenty minutes or we're going to increase cadence, I tell them to envision climbing a real mountain—after all, they're working just as hard as if they were! If you can make it to the top of this mountain, you can make it through any adversity you face. And you can take it all out on the bike.

I've taught hundreds of Spinning classes, and to this day I look forward to every class. Each ride encapsulates the daily battle to stay fit and focused. Each ride ends in a small personal victory. It reminds me that I am capable of doing anything, as long as I keep going. It also reminds me, on a daily basis, that hard work leads to a sense of achievement and deep satisfaction. Every time I work out, the sacrifice and effort create joy. It's not like you endure the pain to get the joy—they are two parts of the same process.

In previous chapters I've talked about the Five Decisions, which change the way you think about yourself, your health, and your entire life. Once you make the Five Decisions, you will not waver in your commitment, you will learn self-control, and you will take responsibility for your life. This is not a diet or just another fitness program; this is a complete change in the way you live. And there is a crucial spiritual dimension to changing your life. When I decided to reclaim my health, I had to accept the fact that I couldn't do it on my own. I had to turn over my lifelong weight battle to God. Without His help I never could have lost 200 pounds.

When I'm in a Spinning class, I gain strength from other members of the class, from the inspiring music, and from the encouragement of the instructor. I rely on God and others to help me succeed. The same will be true for you. You're about to change your life, so draw strength from God and from other people.

EXCEEDING YOUR DREAMS

A few years into my journey, I started dreaming about running a marathon. I had always thought, *How amazing for your feet to be your transportation.* That concept had not been a part of my life in the past. Once I was fit, though, a marathon seemed like the perfect peak moment to work toward. I had another reason too. My mom was battling leukemia. As I watched her fight the disease, I decided that, rather than sit around feeling helpless, I would raise money for the cause and train with a group for the Disney Marathon. I'll never forget hearing "26.2 miles" and thinking, *How can that be possible?*

The training was unbelievably intense. Harder than I expected. Remember, I live in South Florida, so training for a marathon means running many miles a day in crushing heat and humidity. And no matter how many miles you run in training, no matter how many toenails you lose (I lost eight!), it comes down to race day. I always get to the point where I'm not sure I can run another step. I just pray this happens at mile twenty-four and not mile five. When my legs start to feel really heavy, I start repeating to myself, *Don't stop! You're getting there. One foot in front of the other. You didn't come this far to quit.* I picture dropping out of the race and having to tell people, "My feet hurt, so I just quit." Don't think so. Being uncomfortable is no reason not to do something—that would be selling out.

71

The thing about pain is that it's temporary, whereas the pride of accomplishment is permanent. It's like pregnancy and giving birth. It's uncomfortable and *hurts,* but the unspeakable joy of meeting each of my children in the delivery room somehow transformed the pain into peak moments—all the sweeter because of the anticipation and final arrival. When I feel pain after an incredibly tough run or Spinning session, it reminds me of the great thing I accomplished. And one thing I know from experience is that the pain of regret is far worse than the pain of discipline.

> *The pain of regret is far worse*
> *than the pain of discipline.*

ENJOY YOUR NEW LIFE

One of the great things about any process of positive transformation is that the longer you do it and avoid temptations to quit, the more you have invested in not failing. Every time you stick with it, it becomes easier to decide to stay on track. By the time I ran that first marathon, there was *no way* I was going back to the place of misery I had come from. In the last mile of the race, I pulled out one of the worst "before" pictures of me ever taken. I stared at it and sobbed, letting the feelings of accomplishment and gratitude wash over me. I had come so far. So much effort, discomfort, and hard work had gone into making that moment possible. So many days of dragging myself to training at 4 a.m. I couldn't have celebrated the person I was on the day of the marathon if I hadn't once been the girl in that photo. And that's the lesson I took away from my first race. The effort you put into something doesn't disappear as you expend it. It all goes into a bank, with interest, and a day comes when you get it all back and more in the form of pure joy.

My whole family—including my mom, who was in remission by that time—was waiting at the finish line. I crossed the line and immediately collapsed, full of pride and exhaustion and a thousand other emotions. I didn't know what the future held for me, for my mom, or for anyone, but I knew that day I had given it my best. And believe me, that was one awesome peak moment! My mom cried, we all hugged, and I knew each person was sharing my joy. Not only had I completed my first marathon just four years after weighing 349 pounds, but my mom was there to celebrate with me! I'll never lose the intensity of that moment.

I ran my second marathon three weeks later because it was my thirty-third birthday and because I'd met way too many people who said, "Yeah, I ran a marathon—once." I wanted to avoid that cliché. And I wanted to keep having moments I would remember for the rest of my life.

———

So I ask you again: when was your last peak moment? Forget, for now, any weight issues. Don't let your appearance or embarrassment or feelings of awkwardness limit you. If you're like me, you want to live intensely. You're tired of squandering time. If I've struck a nerve, good. That means you're ready to start your own Brain Change. I believe in you, and I can promise that you'll never be the same.

Never-Say-Diet Tip

Rewards and peak moments are essential to your ongoing success. I recently checked in with a client who had lost 50 pounds in five months and strengthened her muscles considerably. I called her cell, and her young daughter answered the phone. I asked if I could speak to her mom. "Mommy's ice skating," she answered. I screamed into the phone, "She's *what*?" I was so proud of her that I started to cry.

Then my client grabbed the phone, bubbling over with excitement. "You should see my kids hugging me," she said. "I haven't done this in more than twenty years. I can't believe it—I have my life back."

I told her to take a mental picture of that moment—what her kids looked like and exactly what it felt like to be gliding over that ice. Then the next time the workouts got hard—and there had been plenty of moments when she'd told me she didn't think she could go on—she had to picture herself doing something she had thought would never happen again. I wanted her also to remember the pride she had given her children that day.

She has proven to herself that the peak moment of having your life back is worth the work!

Chapter 6

The Five Brain-Change Decisions

Decide Not to Let Life Pass You By!

Making any lasting life change is a process. I wish I could tell you that all you need is a tearful breakdown followed by a sincere prayer and you will instantly achieve all your goals. It is necessary to reach a point where you are no longer willing to continue living the way you have been. And I do believe in the power of prayer. But truthfully, transformation isn't that easy, and it doesn't happen in just a moment.

A big part of the reason that it's hard to achieve lasting

change is that your brain works against you. I'm a prime example. My brain had been conditioned to remember every failure and weakness, to the point that I maintained the habit of always letting myself down. It was years before I realized that to lose weight I had to reprogram my thinking, or any change I achieved wouldn't last. I had to erase some of the old me but at the same time build on my good qualities so I could live a new life with confidence. I needed to personalize the plan.

In retrospect I realize my success was based on five decisions that I made. Those decisions became the gold standard for how I would live from then on. They gave me a foundation for facing tough choices, especially on days when I was tired or had lost my enthusiasm. Anytime the part of me that wanted to cop out would start to gain the upper hand, I would replay the Five Decisions, and they would keep me from letting myself off the hook. These decisions are now part of my core belief system. They keep me forever grounded.

Whether you want to lose 5 pounds or 105 pounds, or whether you're struggling with an entirely different life issue, you need to get serious about reprogramming yourself for long-term success. Fear holds all of us back by keeping our failures close and our dreams distant. The process of physical change takes time, but the good news is that you can overcome your fear of failure by changing your brain with the Five Decisions. Make these decisions today.

> *Fear holds all of us back*
> *by keeping our failures close*
> *and our dreams distant.*

1. BE TRUTHFUL

You have to start here, and I'll warn you: this one can really hurt. The truth is, we all put on different personas in different situations, but you are the only one who knows who you are when no one else is in the room. I've told you what a great actress I was. I had people believing I was confident and happy with my life. No matter how authentic we'd like to be, we keep some things hidden. Especially when it comes to the parts of our lives we don't like. We get really good at hiding disappointment and self-hatred.

We all fail, and nobody wants to wear a sign that says "I blew it again!" The great news is, you can face up to your failures and get rid of a lot of fear by allowing yourself no more excuses. To do that, the first decision you have to make is to be completely honest about your failures. When you change your brain, you begin to identify all the excuses you've been using to sabotage your success. I realized I had always mislabeled my excuses, calling them "reasons" that explained why I had setbacks or couldn't reach a goal. I couldn't begin to change until I abandoned that thinking. Neither can you.

I had to tell myself the truth—that I had been a liar. I know that sounds harsh, but remember, the truth can be hard to take. In the past, whenever I said I didn't have time to exercise, I was really saying that exercise was not important enough to me to make time. Or I'd promise myself I'd give up all sugar on Monday so I could eat an extra piece of birthday cake on Sunday, but by Monday afternoon some stressful event would drive me to the cookie jar. Those lies had to stop.

When I made the first of the Five Decisions, I was done with lying to myself. My first commitment was to tell the truth even when it was painful to do so.

Now, when I speak to groups, I often hand out blank sheets of paper. I ask everyone to write down all the excuses they've used in the past, whether it was an illness, financial stress, a family crisis, or anything else. They keep the list private, and they have to be completely honest with themselves. When they finish, I tell them to hold on to the list as a reminder whenever they are tempted later to give up on achieving their fitness goal. Often I see tears running down their faces.

Owning up to the truth is emotional. It is also the greatest step you can take to get started. So before you read the next section, find your own sheet of paper. Write down your list. Keep it private, but keep it handy to use later when you need a reminder.

2. BE FORGIVING

Some of the greatest success stories of all time have come from people who regularly had failed but remained determined. Thomas Edison endured many failures for every experiment that succeeded, and Lance Armstrong very nearly hung up his biking career after years of disappointing results. Eventually they used their previous failures as motivation for future success.

With the second of the Five Decisions, it's time to pick yourself up, dust yourself off, and look ahead. If you fall back on old habits and remind yourself of all the times you vowed to do something and then failed, you're preparing for yet another failure. Your second decision, to be forgiving, retrains your brain to think differently about who you are.

Negative people have trouble forgiving others and themselves. But you are no longer a negative person, which means you are now free to forgive yourself. Remember, the best example of forgiveness comes from God. We are all guilty of something, whether it's a bad attitude or hurting someone or speaking words that are unkind. I'm way too familiar with my mistakes. But I also know I can ask for forgiveness and choose to be better and try harder, effective immediately. You can do the same thing. You are no longer defined by your past. Move on.

On the other hand—and here is the tough part—forgiveness is not a license for further failure. Forgive yourself, but learn important lessons from your mistakes. You really must be careful not to let the ability to forgive yourself become a new excuse not to get the job done. In other words, get over the past, then get on with your future.

3. BE COMMITTED

Success is a direct result of commitment. We all know this, but we allow fear to convince us we can't make it happen. Often that's because we look too far into the future and tell ourselves we won't be able to keep at it over the long haul. Well, here is some fantastic news: the strength and level of your commitment will grow as the success starts to happen. The important thing is to decide today that you will be committed, and then let the small successes you experience every day build your confidence and commitment.

The decision to stay committed will be easier as you see results and have more and more invested in what you've already accomplished. I have seen this with many of my clients. I'll see the insecurity in their eyes and hear their negative self-talk when I'm trying to rally them for a workout. But with small early successes, their confidence builds, and in just a few weeks, they are excited about long-term success.

For the Brain Change to work for you, you must shift your thinking away from dramatic weight loss and focus on changing the way you think of yourself. You are breaking a bad habit. Therefore, your job in the beginning is to concentrate on sticking to a small goal and then using your growing confidence to achieve more challenging goals. In the beginning I made up my mind to do one thing: I would exercise for thirty minutes a day for one month. I took Sundays off for a mental and physical break. It was challenging yet realistic. By the end of that month, my commitment was more intense, because I was starting to believe in myself. And I wasn't about to quit, because that would have meant I'd wasted the entire month!

My life was changing. I was no longer failing and then lying to myself. I was reprogramming myself by keeping one simple promise at a time.

Prepare yourself for frustration. It's hard to start exercising and not see immediate results. I remember feeling that things were taking too long. When that happened, I had to have a chat with God and give myself lots of positive reinforcement. There was no quick fix, pill, or other program that could deliver what had always been missing before—my unconditional commitment to being done with fat! And this time I was going to do it!

4. Be Interested

When I began my journey, I had no real formula for success in losing weight. I had to be willing to learn, to be a student again. I had to gain an understanding of what works and what doesn't. That meant asking questions as well as doing my own research. It meant being interested in how the human body works.

The fourth decision, being interested, might seem optional. But don't discount its importance. It allows you to take charge of your life and your health. I always think it's hysterical when I see an advertisement that promises "Fast and easy results! We do all the thinking and planning for you!" Oh yeah? Well, where can I find you when I'm on a cruise or at the buffet and the prepackaged, perfectly portioned meal has not been delivered? And come to think of it, why should I be dependent on the diet industry when it's my life?

When you learn on your own to make the right choices, it transforms you. If you hand over these crucial decisions to a diet plan that supplies your food and does the thinking for you, you're giving up control. But when you take the necessary steps to understand how your body works and metabolizes and why exercise is essential, you start to give meaning to all your eating and fitness decisions. It's one thing to be told that skipping breakfast is bad and another to understand that a healthy breakfast fires your metabolism and keeps you energetic and burning calories all day. Everything starts to make sense, and it's a lot easier to make hard choices when you understand why you need to make them.

So, be truthful, be forgiving, be committed, and be interested. Those are the first four crucial decisions you need to make if you want to change your life. Be honest about the old excuses you've relied on. Make an unconditional commitment to work daily and to achieve your long-term goals. Forgive yourself for past failures, and focus firmly on your future success. And take a personal interest in how your body works.

When I first made those decisions, I was almost ready to move forward... but then I realized there was one more, and for me it was the most necessary decision. Ultimately, it was the decision that delivered every success I've had. I never would have lost 200 pounds if I hadn't made the fifth decision: to surrender.

5. SURRENDER

I was so tired of trying and failing to lose weight. I hated that I had no self-worth. I had tried diets and eating plans and exercise, but I'd always tackled it alone. I'd start and quit, then start again later. Or I'd rely on the "experts" to tell me about some trendy new way to make the pounds melt away. I ended up more exhausted and discouraged than when I started. I decided this time had to be different. I had made four crucial decisions, but I needed insurance that I was going to succeed.

Do you really want to win? Are you exhausted from fighting all the up-and-down weight battles? Can you imagine having victory in every area of your life? Wouldn't it be awesome never to worry that you might go back to being the old you? Don't you want to drop the masks and lose the fear and gain confidence and hope?

If that's what you desire (and who doesn't?), here is the fifth decision. It's one you probably don't expect, because it has to do with letting go. True and complete surrender made all the difference for me. I truthfully don't worry any longer about whether I'm going to gain back the weight I lost. Not just because I didn't go on a diet to get here, but because God guaranteed me the victory if I did the work, and He has given me the strength when I didn't have much left.

Alcoholics Anonymous has helped countless people overcome addiction. The twelve-step program begins with reciting the serenity prayer: "God, grant me the serenity to accept the things I cannot change, courage to change the things I can, and the wisdom to know the difference." When a broken person gets to the end of her rope, she is given hope that there is help beyond herself. This can be the basis for overcoming any addiction that is ruining your life.

Our weight, our bodies, our food issues—these are all things we have the power to change! Yet none of us has the strength to do it alone, which is why surrendering—ending the solo battle and beginning afresh—is the answer. God will grant us the power if we do the work.

When I reached the point of desperation, I decided that my new life would be one of striving each day to be the best I could be. And as I surrendered the old miserable me, God gave me the strength to press on. It worked when I began, and it still works, especially on the dark days. Can you fully surrender too? You have decided to do what it takes to change your life. You're committed, but you can't do this alone. Surrender to God, ask Him to help you, and then trust Him to be there for you.

IT'S TIME TO DECIDE

These are the Five Decisions:
1. Be Truthful
2. Be Forgiving
3. Be Committed
4. Be Interested
5. Surrender

If you want to establish a foundation that will support your success for the rest of your life, these are the decisions you have to make. Life change will not be permanent without them. And now, if you have made the Five Decisions, it's time to get to work. Breaking the fat habit for good is going to take determination, but it will happen for you just as it did for me. It is within your reach to never need to say diet again.

For the next sixteen weeks you will need to give me your full and unconditional attention. After that, you will be transformed—and on your own. You will have changed your brain—your attitude about yourself, your approach to failure, and your bedrock commitment to a new life. At the end of sixteen weeks—not all that long when you think about it—you may not have reached your ultimate weight goal, but you will be well on your way to health and fitness. And you will have the confidence it takes to stick with it for good. Your success will continue.

Step by step, without gimmicks or unrealistic promises, we will begin a journey together that will be the start of a new life, not a new diet! It's important that you laugh along the way, enjoy each small success, and get excited about this. It's an adventure, and it takes a lot of passion. But that's what keeps

Don't Hold Back!

Getting good at anything, including exercise, takes practice as well as a willingness to put yourself out there. So stop worrying about timing or circumstances or what others might think of you.

I'll never forget the time I took my son Jake shopping with me at Home Depot. He was two years old and working on potty training at the time. I was looking at lighting fixtures, and I didn't notice that he had slipped away. When I realized it, I looked around, and there was Jake with a crowd around him. He was naked and proudly peeing into a display toilet! I couldn't help but laugh.

Like Jake, you gotta seize the moment! I challenge you just to go for it, like my son—well, maybe not quite like that. Without the usual self-consciousness we all possess, take charge and make disciplined exercise happen in your life, no matter what.

it interesting and enjoyable. We'll make the challenging things in life fun! And you *are* going to have fun—that I promise you.

But here's another promise. No matter how excited you are about doing this, the pressures and demands of life will try to rob you of that excitement nearly every day. I found that out quickly when my husband lost his job and my mom had a relapse of leukemia. However, this time I had asked God to be my strength—and I meant it, which I had failed to do in my previous attempts to lose weight. I found that before I got going each day, I needed to pledge not to let myself get distracted. So I created a Surrender Statement that I repeated as often as I needed to:

> I surrender today. I am going to be the best I can be! I will not let the frustration of trying to wear so many hats take over this mission, no matter what happens. I will respect my body today. I know it is a gift. Thank You, God, for being my strength.

If you are simply trying to lose 10 pounds and get fit, you might not need to repeat the Surrender Statement. But if you've been fighting a losing battle with your weight for years, if you are setting out to change your life for good, consider creating a Surrender Statement of your own, and repeat it each morning to keep yourself on track. Your responsibilities, roles, goals, and beliefs may be different than mine, so make it personal and memorize it. It doesn't need to be fancy, just sincere.

MY SURRENDER STATEMENT

THE BRAIN-CHANGE CONTRACT

You have read and given serious consideration to the Five Decisions that spark the Brain Change. Having made those decisions, you now have a tool for staring down failure and lighting the fire of fearlessness in your life! But before you begin Phase 1 (in the next chapter), understand that committing to a fit and focused life is not like committing to a thirty-day diet. You are committing to a completely different lifestyle. It's going to test you—count on it! There will be times when it will be much more convenient to neglect the program for a couple of days. But don't even consider that possibility.

When you take this step to change your life, there is no going back. You are making a promise to yourself, and you can't back out later—so put it in writing.

A contract is a serious thing. You are giving your word. And remember, you have already decided to stop lying to yourself. While this agreement is for you alone, find someone to witness it for you. That will make you accountable to someone else, as I was with my husband when I began this new way of living. Read the contract, but please don't sign it unless you are ready so it has a lasting effect. Later, whenever you need to, pull it out, look at your signature, remember the day when you asked your witness to add his or her signature, and most of all recall the sincerity in your heart to always be the best you can be.

Note: I meet people almost every day who are already pretty good at exercise, yet they still struggle constantly with their weight. If this describes your experience, you know how frustrating it can be. The good news is that the Brain-Change program will work for you beautifully. If you have an exercise habit that includes at least thirty minutes of a cardiovascular workout five days a week, then begin the program in Phase 2. This is where the nutrition changes take place and the strength training begins. Let's take the discipline you already have and let it spill over into your eating habits. Then watch the transformation!

The Brain-Change Challenge Contract

I, _____, am ready to work hard and to keep at it when circumstances work against me. I will take control of my food issues once and for all and will focus on my optimal health and fitness. By signing this contract, I am making an unconditional commitment to God, myself, and those who love and care about me. I will give my best every day.

From now on I will be *truthful*, even when it hurts. I will stop buying my old excuses—they will no longer hold me back from becoming the person I want to be. I will also be *forgiving* of my past. I accept that I have been slacking in some areas, but I am now done living with disappointment. I am ready to be totally *committed* to creating a new life, no matter what curve balls life throws my way. In order to do this forever, I will take responsibility by understanding the way my body is designed to function. I will be *interested* in nutrition and exercise, and I will try to love it.

I accept that this is going to be difficult some days and that at times I will be frustrated and uncomfortable. However, I also know that doing anything great and worthwhile requires patience, perseverance, and endurance. This is also what makes us "great"! I agree to complete cardiovascular exercise five days a week and to progress into a strength-training program as well. I choose to stop living to eat and start eating to live. I understand that sacrifice and going to bed hungry some nights are what it will take to lose the weight that has been weighing down my life. As I attain my goals, I will continue to put premium food into my body so that I have the best fuel possible to operate on. By living according to this agreement, I will put an end to the old me. I have a new brain. With God's help and my unconditional commitment, I am done fighting this war! I completely and enthusiastically *surrender*!

Signed: _____

Date: _____

Witness: _____

PART TWO

······

Act

Chapter 7

Phase 1
Get a Move On!

Weeks 1–4

Your Goal:
to establish a regular exercise habit.

What You'll Need to Have
- A digital scale
- Clothes to sweat in
- A good attitude about exercise—come on, it's only thirty minutes!
- A plastic tape measure

What You'll Need to Know
- Why cardiovascular exercise is the place to start
- Why eating breakfast is so important

- How to take your measurements
- The math of losing weight

What You'll Need to Do
- Start the day with your Surrender Statement.
- Choose which exercises will work best for you.
- Complete thirty minutes of exercise per day, five days in a row, each week for four weeks, no matter what!
- Eat breakfast, whether you feel like it or not.
- Begin taking your measurements.
- Treat this like the job you've wanted to land as long as you can remember.

———

You are ready for day one of the Brain Change. In the first four weeks, all you need to do is establish discipline and a routine. Forget what you've tried in the past. This is a brand-new start. For now, forget about menus, counting calories, good carbs, bad fats, and whole grains. The goal for Phase 1 is to establish discipline in an exercise program. The root problem of most people who have failed to lose weight and keep it off is not a lack of desire or sincerity but a lack of well-rooted discipline. That's why this program begins with discipline.

Discipline is a learned behavior pattern; it doesn't come naturally. I spent years wishing I had it. I envied those who did, sure that they had been born with some magical gene. These people usually looked great from head to toe and had perfectly organized closets and spotless minivans with the CDs in little baskets, and their favorite pastime was scrapbooking. And those were just my friends who were moms. Then there were my single girlfriends, who managed to work fifty hours a week, take a step-aerobics class, run a 5K on the weekend for breast-cancer research, and always wear the latest fashions. I felt inadequate.

I hid my low self-esteem by telling myself I lived in the moment, always putting others' needs first. But that was a fancy way of disguising the truth that I wasn't willing to do the things that bored me or made me uncomfortable, even if they would cause me to be more organized, healthier, and happier. The people who seemed to be more together were willing to be inconvenienced and to set aside certain things to accomplish the important things. They maintained their focus and found time to work toward achieving their goals, while I was probably baking a cake and watching *Melrose Place*. We had different priorities.

I don't have any more discipline than other people, even though I have lost 200 pounds and can run 26.2 miles. I succeeded because I finally committed to regularly doing things that made me uncomfortable, and I did them long enough that I became comfortable doing them. I changed the way I think so that I became reprogrammed to enjoy exercise and healthy eating. My priorities changed, partly because I got a better sense of what was at stake.

> *I succeeded because I finally committed to regularly doing things that made me uncomfortable, and I did them long enough that I became comfortable doing them.*

DO THIS FOR THOSE YOU LOVE

We all get excited when we think about dropping five dress sizes, but being overweight is much more serious than that. It can kill you. Being overweight is a factor in 14 to 20 percent of cancer deaths. An estimated ninety thousand cancer deaths each year could be avoided if every American maintained a healthy weight.[3] Being overweight also increases the risk of strokes and heart attacks, which kill hundreds of thousands of people each year. This is not to scare you but to educate you. For me, grasping the health aspect of exercise was crucial, because I had denied the danger for so many years. Plus, many of the leading weight-loss programs don't stress the health benefits of losing weight. "Just eat our food and watch the fat melt away"—that's what I'm always hearing. But losing a few dress sizes is only a small part of changing your life.

Your entire success on my program comes from becoming ferociously consistent about exercise. Can you handle that? I know I sound like a drill sergeant, but the exercise component must become as automatic as brushing your teeth. Some programs prescribe two or three days a week of exercise, maybe because it sounds doable. In my experience, if the goal is three days per week, it will be too easy to take days off. The week starts out well. You work out Monday, take off Tuesday because you'll get in Wednesday and Friday, but then you miss Wednesday, so you've got Thursday, but you forgot you had a meeting on Thursday. Before you know it, it's Friday, and you've worked out only once, and the weekend is conveniently booked up. You have negotiated and not exercised. Exercise needs to become part of your routine—five days a week.

In Phase 1 you will develop a new pattern. Five days in a row you will break a sweat with thirty minutes of cardiovascular exercise. Period. When I started, I committed to six days a week and took Sundays off. But I don't think that was necessary. Five days is better to get the full benefits yet avoid burnout or injury. And you can pick the time of day that's best for you to exercise. The important thing is to get started and get moving. So pick a time, choose an exercise you don't hate, and decide how intense you want it to be. Just make it happen.

If you find that you miss a day or two, it's no big deal. Don't let a minor thing become a discouraging failure. Simply begin again with a new day one, and get a fresh start. Don't think of starting over as punishment; it just means you'll devote a few extra weeks to completing Phase 1. You need to stick to thirty minutes a day, five days a week, for four consecutive weeks to develop your new habit. There's no point in going on to Phase 2 until your cardio routine is as regular as the mail. If you aren't willing to do that, then *put down this book right now!* This program can't help you until you have established a new discipline in your life. (And remember, whenever you start a new exercise program, first get a physical examination from your doctor.)

CUSTOMIZE YOUR PROGRAM

Just to show you that I'm not a drill sergeant, I'll say this: exercise is exercise. Convenience can be an important factor both in getting started and in sticking with it. If you have time to hike in the mountains for thirty minutes, great. If you want to run on a treadmill in your bedroom while watching television, that's fine too. It all works. But if it takes you forty-five minutes to get to the mountains just to begin your hike, you might find that an exercise that minimizes commuting time will keep you more motivated.

For many people, going to a gym really does make the most sense. One benefit is the great variety of exercise options. You can try out a number of different machines and discover what you like and don't like. Even the act of walking into a health club can serve as a useful transition from the outside world to your thirty minutes of exercise. It helps you focus—you are there for one reason only. A health club can even be a great support system as you meet other people who share the common goal of becoming fit. But I also understand that a lot of people are intimidated by the gym environment. All I can say is, if I could get comfortable in a gym, anybody can!

I made one of my first visits to a gym because I had received an invitation in the mail for a free training session. I weighed well over 300 pounds. I showed up for my appointment, excited and nervous, thinking, *This could be it!* The trainer admitted that this was only his third day on the job, which actually reassured me. We were both learning something new.

He said we needed to establish my body-fat percentage. He handed me a fancy, hand-held electronic device I'd never seen before—and I'm not sure he had either. He entered certain data, including my age, gender, and a weight that I grossly underestimated, and told me to grip the device in my hand and within a few seconds we'd have our answer. I held on tight as the machine attempted to calculate a number. A few seconds later, it read ERROR. Great. "Oh well," I said. But he insisted we try again. Same thing: ERROR. I was ready to run out the door and never look back, but he wouldn't let up until we did it a *third* time, and of course it said the same thing: ERROR.

He began rummaging through his desk for the manual. I just wanted to

Never-Say-Diet Tip

Consistency without excuses is what forms new habits. A day will come—probably in your second week, because the first week you'll be pumped up—when the whole day slides by, and you still haven't done your exercise. That is the crisis moment. Will you still squeeze it in? Those days happened to me, and you know what I did? At ten o'clock at night, I'd put on my watch, head out the door, and circle my cul-de-sac for thirty minutes. I knew I wasn't going to have the workout of my life, but it didn't matter. I had to show up. I now know those times were critical in making me tough enough to see this through. I didn't want to drag myself out the door late at night, but I did it anyway. Embrace those willpower challenges when they occur; they are helping you forge unbreakable habits!

die and leave my body there. He finally found the instructions and searched the troubleshooting section, locating the notes regarding the ERROR message. Then moving his finger over to the explanation column and reading out loud, he said, "More than 50 percent body fat. Can't calculate accurately."

Yes, I was so fat that the machine couldn't work. And now this nice trainer got to experience my humiliation with me. He tried to make me feel better. He smiled and said, "That's okay. We're gonna fix that!" I sat through his introduction to working out and left, just another day in workout paradise. But I used my feelings of discomfort to my advantage. I showed up again and again, determined to make the next time different.

You need to make the same commitment: this time is going to be different!

Choosing an Exercise

When I started exercising, I needed a low-impact activity. I didn't want to get an injury as soon as I started. At first I used a recumbent bike, which I recommend, especially if you're seriously overweight. You sit in a normal, chair-like seat on a recumbent bike, which takes pressure off your tailbone. You can go at any speed you want, and you can increase resistance gradually.

With that as one option, remember that the most important criterion for choosing an exercise is that it is something you will keep doing. You can pick a few different exercises and rotate them to keep things fresh, or you can find one you really like and stick with it. Either way, make sure you exercise every day, five days in a row, each week for four weeks, without exception.

The amount of calories you will burn will vary, depending on a number of factors, including your size, your lean-muscle mass, your metabolic rate, the exercise you choose, and the intensity of your activity. Exercise that requires more movement will burn more calories. For now, though, don't key in on how many calories you're burning. Your objective in Phase 1 is to establish discipline and a routine. Showing up is the main thing. Choose an exercise based on what you like and what is convenient. Here are some suggestions. They all work, but remember, to qualify as exercise, they need to raise your heart rate and breathing. (This means you, walkers!)

Brisk walking	Swimming
Jogging/running	Tennis
Bike riding	Basketball
Stationary bike / recumbent bike	Racquetball
Elliptical machine	Spinning class
Cross-country skiing machine	Step aerobics
Stair climber	Kick boxing
Stair stepper	Dancing

Don't Skip Breakfast

You do have one other task this month. Simply start each day by eating breakfast. For the majority of overweight people I've known, including the old me, breakfast is the meal they most likely skip. Big mistake. A recent Harvard study found that people who eat breakfast have only half the risk of being overweight or developing diabetes compared to people who skip breakfast.[4] An ongoing study conducted by the National Weight Control Registry found that people who have lost at least 30 pounds and kept it off for a year or more regularly eat breakfast. Among the nearly three thousand men and women enrolled in the research, 78 percent cited eating breakfast every day as one of their strategies.[5]

It's no surprise why. When you don't give your body any fuel in the morning, it starts to slow down and conserve energy. You creep through the day, burning fewer calories than normal. When you fuel up in the morning, however, your body runs at high energy all day. Whether you are hungry or not, give your body something to run on at the beginning of your day. Even if you are a breakfast hater, make sure you eat something before starting the day.

Taking Your Measurements

A scale tells only part of the story. You will want to track your measurements as well so you can stay motivated when the scale isn't being your friend. Taking your measurements now allows you to see exactly how much is coming off later and from where. As you build muscle, there may be months where your progress shows more dramatically in your measurements than in your weight, because muscle weighs more than fat. Also, the health benefits of weight loss apply primarily to fat lost from the abdomen. If the number on your scale isn't declining rapidly, but your waist has lost several inches and your jeans are looser, you can rest assured that you're making improvement!

When you measure yourself, make sure you keep up with six measurements. You should be able to do five of them by yourself using a plastic tape measure. To take your arm measurement, don't hesitate to ask a friend or your spouse to help. Having a partner can be a great source of encouragement along the way and can provide some valuable accountability.

As you measure, remember to keep your muscles relaxed and to pull the tape measure to a natural tightness. Be sure you consistently measure in the same spots. I also recommend doing this before your workouts.

1. Bust
Without squishing, measure all the way around your back and bust at the nipple line, not lower.

2. Chest
Measure under your breasts, but as high as you can go, making sure the tape is straight as you go all the way around your back.

3. Upper Arms
Measure where they are the biggest, above your elbows.

4. *Waist*

Measure wherever your waist is the smallest. If you have no defined waistline, go around the navel line.

5. *Hips*

Measure at the biggest part, even if it seems close to the top of your thighs.

6. *Thighs*

Measure where they are the biggest.

DOING THE MATH

I know, I know, I promised to keep the math to a minimum. And I will. But part of taking charge of your weight and fitness is getting a handle on how much stuff you should be stuffing in your body—and how fast you can expect to see the extra weight disappear once you change the energy equation. Trust me, this is math you're going to like. And it won't require any calculators!

To know how much food you should eat on any given day, you need to know how many calories a day your body burns. Remember, to lose weight, your goal is to use more calories each day than you consume, because then your body will generate extra fuel from your fat stores. Think of it like a bank account. When you deposit more than you use, your body stores the excess as a "savings account" in the form of fat. When you spend more energy than you've deposited, it's like spending more money than you've earned—your body needs to draw on the savings account to make up the difference. It starts liquidating your fat supplies and burning them for energy.

Your body uses a certain number of calories each day simply maintaining itself—breathing, pumping blood, digesting food, blinking, thinking, and using all those tiny involuntary muscles we never even notice. That's what we call *resting metabolism.*

Overall, an average-sized woman—five feet four inches tall and 145 pounds—burns about 1,200 calories per day just living a normal life—sleeping, eating, driving to work or school or church, walking across a few parking lots, cooking meals, and so on. Some additional walking occurs as part of a normal day, and maybe an occasional set of stairs gets climbed, but that's all the physical activity that's included in this resting metabolism number. Smaller women will burn less energy, larger women more. A tall, overweight woman might burn 2,000 calories per day.

Any additional activity uses more energy and burns additional calories. So if the average woman walks for an hour, she might burn an extra 300 calories, meaning she burns a total of 1,500 that day. If she eats 1,500 calories' worth of food, she's energy (and weight) balanced. If she eats more than that, her body will take the extra food, break it down, convert it to fat, and store it on her body. That's what fat is—a concentrated form of energy, conveniently stored on your thighs for when it's needed! It's a good system. If you couldn't store extra energy before you actually need it, then anytime your body used up whatever food you'd put into it, you would keel over like a switched-off toy.

So the key to weight loss is to push your daily "burn" well beyond your daily intake. How much? Well, it differs from person to person. It depends on how much weight you want to lose, how intense you want to be about exercising, and what your body's natural set point is. Some people's bodies resist weight loss more than others. But the rule of thumb is that every 10-calorie shift in the daily energy equation will result in a 1-pound weight shift over a year. So if every day you burn 300 more calories than you eat, you will lose 30 pounds in a year. On the other hand, if you eat 100 more calories per day than you burn, you will gain 10 pounds in that year.

Another way to think of it is to know that you must burn 3,500 calories more than you eat to lose a pound. If your goal is to lose 1 pound a week, that's 500 calories a day—which is about how much you'll burn doing the exercises in this program. Combine that with healthy eating, and you can exceed 1 pound a week.

Okay, math lesson over! Now that wasn't so bad, was it?

• • • • • •

How Cardio Works

Cardiovascular exercise is simply fitness training for your heart—the most important muscle in your body. You get only one, and it is literally what keeps you running. Due to our desk jobs and modern lifestyles, we don't get enough daily training for the heart anymore. So we must schedule it.

Here's how it works. When you start exercising, your muscles need fuel to keep going and oxygen to burn that fuel—just like your car. Your lungs work to breathe in more oxygen during the activity, and your heart works to pump oxygen and fuel through your bloodstream and into your muscles so you can continue. This process conditions the heart by making it work hard and then recover, so it becomes stronger and more efficient. The more regular and intense your workouts become, the better your heart operates.

As your heart becomes more efficient, you lower your resting heart rate, which is the number of beats per minute it takes for your heart to keep you alive when you are at rest. A strong, well-conditioned heart can pump more blood with every beat, so it doesn't have to beat as often. This can save a lot of wear and tear. A poorly conditioned person's resting heart rate might be eighty beats per minute, while a fit person's might be sixty beats per minute. Saving that extra twenty beats per minute, to do the same job, can add a lot of extra hours, days, and years to your heart's life span.

The more fit you become, the greater endurance you have. And more endurance means you are using more fuel, which comes from the food you consume—or consumed in the past! You burn more calories—in other words, you lose weight.

A body that gets used to burning lots of calories during exercise also burns more calories when at rest. That's what we call *metabolism*—the rate at which your body burns calories, both while you're hanging out and working out. When you get out of breath during the exercise, that's your body trying to use oxygen it doesn't have. The more fit you are, the better your body gets at running an oxygen deficit and making up for it later. After a good run, while you're at home watching television, your body is still working hard to get oxygen and energy slotted back into your muscles for the next exertion. We call this the *after burn,* and it can burn lots of calories—for up to fifteen hours after a challenging workout.

For those reasons and more, cardiovascular exercise is the best way to start your program. Here is what it provides you:

- stronger heart
- weight loss by burning calories both during and after the workout
- reduced chance of heart attack and stroke
- improved blood pressure and cholesterol and blood-sugar levels
- improved moods, reduced stress level, and less depression
- improved sleep
- decreased body fat, improved immune function, increased endurance and energy
- improved confidence and contentment

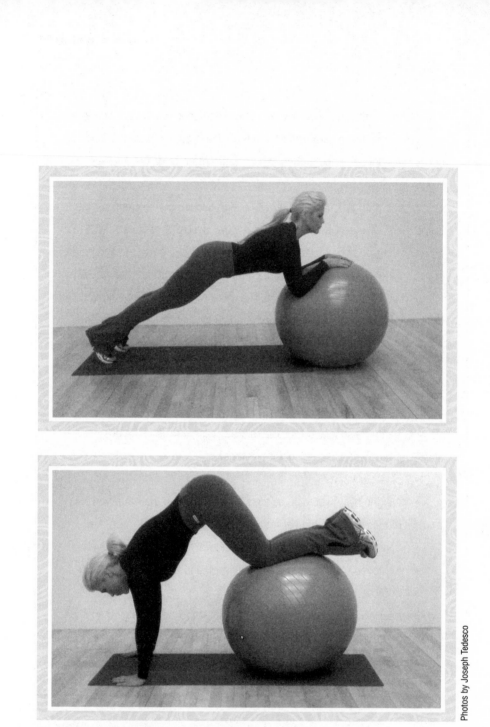

Some days I still can't believe I can do this stuff!

Chapter 8

Phase 2
Take Charge!

Weeks 5–8

Your Goal:
to regain control of what you choose to put into your mouth, on your own terms!

What You'll Need to Have
- A stability ball that fits you

What You'll Need to Know
- Why strength training is essential
- Why liquid calories are many people's downfall

What You'll Need to Do
- Start the day with your Surrender Statement.

- Continue the same cardio plan: five days per week, thirty minutes per day.
- Introduce strength training on the stability ball: two days per week, twenty minutes per day.
- Choose your food weak spot, and stay away from it for a month.
- Keep a log of your weekly weight and measurements (recorded on the same day and time each week).
- Keep a food journal so you can see what you are actually eating every day.

Congratulations! You've stuck to the Phase 1 plan and exercised faithfully for the past month. You're developing a healthy routine and the discipline that will carry you through. For me, part of the excitement was being able to say, "Yeah, I work out," and having it be the truth.

Phase 2 begins today. It's where you solidify your new habit while introducing strength training and making some changes to what you eat and drink. Remember, the program builds gradually with each phase so you will succeed in making changes that stick.

When I began this program, a regimented meal plan would have freaked me out. Instead, I gradually reestablished my relationship with food. To do that, I knew exactly where to start. (And you probably know where I'm headed.)

My weak spot was sugar and snacks, really all processed junk food. That had to go. During Phase 2, I still ate my favorite meals, but they couldn't include sweets, candy, or chips—not even the pretzels that smelled so good in the mall. I figured I could give up the snacks I loved, which were doing nothing for me nutritionally, as long as I still had something to look forward to, like steak, chicken cordon bleu, and maybe pizza. I wasn't ready to embrace unfamiliar foods, but I was ready to eliminate the obvious junk.

I'll never forget the first day of Phase 2. I had a big challenge. My friend LeeAnn had invited me to a Princess House crystal party—like a Tupperware party, only with fancier stuff for the kids to break. I knew there'd be desserts, but I couldn't back out of the party, so I showed up after dinner and sat down to what would have been a dream for me in the past; only now it was a nightmare. Every homemade cookie recipe I loved had been made. I sat there and started to shake. *I did say I was going to ease my way into this... Total deprivation isn't necessary, is it?... Better to indulge myself ever so slightly, then go cold turkey tomorrow... What's one cookie, right?*

Wrong! I knew myself too well! One cookie would have meant a second cookie and perhaps even a third. I had not yet broken my addiction to sugar. Thank God I came to my senses before I reached for that first cookie. I had made a promise to myself, and a promise is a promise. I had to be strong this time. One cookie was never one cookie for me. And even if it was only this night, I had already drawn clear lines, and that little cookie would cross it.

I did it. I left that night without eating a crumb, and as soon as I got into the car, I realized I had just had a small victory. The power to say no and deal with temptation was inside me after all. I had taken a major step toward gaining control over my life. I just needed to practice and remember from then on how good I felt that night.

I also resolved to give up all liquid calories during the month of Phase 2. (If you're thinking along these lines, this applies to fruit juice, soft drinks, and alcohol.) It was another way to cut some calories from my life with little sacrifice. I occasionally drank diet drinks but stuck to water as much as possible.

As I trained my mind not to give in to cravings while still enjoying food, a funny thing happened. After the first week of Phase 2, I found myself eating smaller meals, even a little healthier. It just felt wrong to stop putting junk into my body and then to overeat at mealtime. Especially with all the exercising I was doing.

Toward the end of that first week we had dinner at an Italian restaurant,

DiSalvos, one of our family's favorite places. I ordered the fettuccine alfredo. When the plate came, I looked at it and knew it was way too much. So I asked for a salad plate and cut the serving in half, putting the rest aside. I ate the half that remained on my plate, and it was delicious. But having a few more bites seemed like a good idea since I was enjoying it so much. Immediately, just like the cookie incident, I had a chat with myself. I resolved that I was finished with dinner and had to put down the fork. I did! Again, another victory. *Keep it up,* I thought. This approach worked well for the next several weeks, and I was proud every time I succeeded.

Start listening to what you tell yourself. Your self-talk is far more powerful than you imagine. If you tell yourself that being hungry is a bad thing, then you're not going to achieve your goals. If you whisper to yourself that you deserve some dessert, prepare for a long, uphill climb. Part of forming new habits is changing the things you tell yourself. Gear your self-talk toward achievement, confidence, and success, and you'll notice that developing discipline is a lot easier than you imagined.

Looking back, the simple act of telling myself I didn't need any more fettuccine was a big step toward making the complete Brain Change. I was choosing to have power over food. I was taking responsibility for my life, and I began seeing results as the readout on the digital scale started to go down.

You aren't at the mercy of your stomach's cravings. Some call this willpower; I call it brain power!

Beginning Phase 2

This is going to be one of the best months of your life. And it will be challenging, because you are going to take charge! Part of taking charge is deciding what to zero in on. I can't tell you what your particular weak spot is—it has to be on your own terms. I can't be there to make sure you cut back and say no to dessert or a high-calorie drink. It's up to you to discover that you aren't at the mercy of your stomach's cravings. Some call this willpower; I call it brain power!

Your first task is to decide what your big downfall is, foodwise, and then resolve to give it up. For you, it's Lent all month long! And this is a more important step than you may realize. No, simply targeting one area of food weakness will not make you fit overnight, but you're making significant progress. Cutting back always hurts a little at first. But it's a terrific mental practice. (In Phase 5 you will learn how to gradually reintroduce some of what you are giving up now.)

In Phase 2 you're responsible for coming up with your own sacrifices, but I'll give you some examples. If junk food is your thing, then don't mess too much with the foods you eat at breakfast, lunch, and dinner. You can start right now to make an impact on your waistline by steering clear of the Krispy Kremes and syrupy latte grandes.

If going back for seconds, thirds, and fourths is your downfall, then that's your target. It's okay to savor the waffles, cobb salads, and cheeseburgers for another month; just reduce your portions. Be sure to walk away from each meal wanting a little more. You will train your stomach to get used to less food at mealtime, while training your brain to take over when it needs to. Some great tricks to help make this happen are to use smaller plates and to drink a glass of water after you finish a meal. The best advice I can offer is to determine the amount you will eat before you take the first bite. Put a sensible portion on your plate, then put the rest away. Don't leave a serving bowl within reach. When you've eaten what's on your plate, that's it. So chew well!

For the sugar fiend, all candy, desserts, cookies, even diet ice cream should be banished this month. It all feeds your craving for sugar, and you must let it go. For the crunch fiend, the same goes for chips and processed snacks. You can still snack, but snack on fresh vegetables (a healthy crunch!), some fruit in the morning, or popcorn (no butter!). One of my clients now insists that frozen grapes are better than cheesecake! Ironically, after a few weeks without much sugar, the fruit will seem sweeter to you than before. You will have reset your taste buds for a new treat.

In this phase, making a major dietary concession is nonnegotiable to your transformation. If you're not ready to take this step, then hang back in Phase 1 until you are. Taking control of food must be a lasting change, not another diet. If you view the lifestyle changes that come in Phase 2 as optional, you shouldn't be here yet. Remember, you've decided to tell yourself the truth. Care enough to be honest about what you're ready for. There is no point in doing this halfway.

Part of your commitment to truth is tracking what you eat this month. A food journal can be very revealing, since many of us have a habit of forgetting lots of the "little things" we put in our mouths over the course of the day. Keep a small notepad with you, and record everything you eat and drink. It's important that you write it down each time you consume something. If you wait until the end of the day, your food record won't be completely accurate.

No matter what eating habit you're working on, stop drinking your calo-

Never-Say-Diet Tip

You might be surprised that I'm not having you launch a strict new eating plan this month. You can if you want, but don't forget that you aren't trying a new diet. You are changing your eating patterns and life habits forever. Don't worry about hitting a certain weight before bathing-suit season; it's far more important that you make small changes over time so the pattern lasts into all the rest of the bathing-suit seasons of your life.

ries. The average American drinks 450 calories a day. That's a needless calorie intake that can add up to a lot of extra pounds each year. If you already drink a protein shake in the morning, continue with that. A shake with lots of protein powder and a little fresh fruit is an excellent breakfast. Pure fruit smoothies, however, are tremendously high in sugar. A twenty-ounce soda contains 250 calories of nutritionless sugar water. Drink two of those a day, and you've had a third of your daily calories—and without any food! What about fruit juice? It has just as many calories as soda. The same is true of beer, wine, and mixed drinks. Sweetened teas and coffees have nearly as many. If you are serious about making a dent in your daily calorie intake, liquid calories are a great place to start.

The worst thing about liquid calories is that they don't make a dent in your hunger. People who drink three colas are just as hungry as people who drink water. Hungrier, perhaps, because they are hooked on having that sweet taste in their mouth. (I admit, however, I do like diet sodas. I try to limit myself to one a day, because I am concerned about the long-term effects of too many sugar substitutes.)

As a way of kicking the sugary soda habit, substituting diet sodas or drinks like Crystal Light can help. If you are even remotely serious about improving your diet—and I know you are, since you and I are working through Phase 2—eliminating sugar from your drinks should be at the top of your agenda. And if you have an occasional glass of wine or other alcoholic beverage, keep in mind that every bottle of beer or glass of wine is approximately 150 calories, and that adds up fast. So drink water instead.

If you are using diet drinks as a transition from sugary drinks, see if you can gradually transition to water. Drinking glasses of clean, cold water throughout the day will keep your energy high and prevent dehydration. In one study in Germany, people who drank two glasses of water immediately raised their metabolisms by 30 percent.[6] I don't care if you drink tap, bottled, or sparkling; all I care is that you get started today.

STRENGTH TRAINING

I can't begin to guess how many people have told me that strength training scares them. That never surprises me, because it scares me too! Gyms seem to have an invisible line running down the middle. On one side is the cardio crowd: the overweight people working hard to lose pounds and the addicts gazing at the readout of calories they are burning. The other side, the weight-room, is where the "serious" people hang out, the ones with rippling muscles and intense focus. At least that's how I'd always seen it before, and even after, I started my own weight training. I figured I had no business over there because I had no clue what to do and it would be embarrassing to try. Also because I was reading the minds of the "gym rats." Their look seemed to be saying, "Go away. Get back on the treadmill where you belong." That held me back for a while, until I discovered that the problem was in my head. I had as much reason to do strength training as anyone else. I would also end up learning a lot from being there.

My hope is that preconceived notions of strength training won't hold you back, because strength training is essential to your long-term goals. The cardio you've been doing is taking great care of your heart and burning lots of calories, but it isn't doing much to build muscle or improve your balance and bone strength. That happens with strength training. Don't be intimidated by that term; it doesn't automatically mean bench presses or the clean and jerk. Strength training is simply any exercise that tests your muscles' strength rather than their endurance, as cardio does.

Muscle is active tissue, so it constantly uses calories for energy to work, repair, and refuel. (Fat, on the other hand, just sits in your body taking up space.) With the aging process—starting as early as our twenties!—we lose muscle, about a pound a year at first. Your calorie needs decrease as this is happening, which means it becomes easier to gain weight. Some of you know this firsthand, because you eat the same way you did ten years ago yet can't stop putting on extra pounds. That's because as you slowly lose muscle, your resting metabolic rate declines. Think of a lake where the same amount of water keeps flowing in at one end, but a little less flows out the other end: the lake gets bigger.

By engaging in regular strength training, you build and replace muscle,

If You Could Feel What I'm Feeling...

In general I think fathers in delivery rooms should speak as little as possible—even a whisper is a reminder that they helped put you in this position. I don't think my father-in-law, Ken, had ever been told this. As Linda, my mother-in-law, was giving birth to her youngest son, Ken sat by, waiting. Linda was in the most intense part of the process, huffing and puffing and giving her all to get that baby out, when the doctor came in, did a check, and announced that the baby would arrive soon. That's when Ken found the need to speak up. "Poor thing," he said, "she can't take much pain."

I wish I could have seen the looks the doctor, nurses, and especially Linda gave him. Fortunately, it was such a ridiculous thing to say that Ken and Linda both still joke about it. But the lesson is this: no one else knows what you're going through right now. Getting through difficult days may be painful, but the rewards later on will make you forget it. This month will be a challenge as you make sacrifices, but that makes it important. Even if people around you won't understand all your emotions, this is your chance to get stronger. And as the challenges come, don't forget to pray.

halting and even reversing the natural muscle decline. More muscle means an increased resting metabolic rate—with more calories burned every single day. I've said a million times to clients, "Cardio burns calories for today; strength training burns them for tomorrow!" You need both for true fitness.

Want more reasons to do strength training? Your muscles are connected to your bones, and by using resistance to train those muscles, you train your bones too. The pull of your muscles on your bones signals your body to reinforce their strength with extra calcium, helping fight osteoporosis and arthritis. And let's not forget that muscle is just prettier than fat. As you become leaner and lighter, you will look much better because of strength training!

BEGIN WITH CORE TRAINING

Most strength-training programs introduce traditional body-part training—you know, biceps curls, chest presses, and so on. But we will start by building and strengthening your core. You need a strong foundation to support additional training, and the body's core muscles are that foundation. They are the muscles deep within the torso. They are attached to your spine and pelvis, and they support the muscles attached to your shoulders too. Keep in mind that your trunk is the main support for your body weight.

Because core training is designed to stretch and strengthen the muscles, tendons, and ligaments that support your spine, it can correct your posture and prevent injuries to your back. By using many muscles to coordinate a movement rather than isolating a single muscle, you will be making the most of your workout time as well.

To do core training, you will use a stability ball, but the secret to its success is actually its instability. When you sit down on one of those big machines at the gym and strap yourself in, you get a lot of artificial support. Machines require no balance, just a fixed motion in one direction. That's great if your goal is to do those machines really well. But your goal is to train your muscles for the complexities of real life—for yard work, carrying in groceries, picking up your kids and swinging them around. That's why we begin with movement training instead of body-part training. In real life you don't lift things with the benefit of sitting still or having something like a bench to support you. Because a stability ball is round and unstable, you need to use your center of gravity—your core—to keep from rolling off. Likewise, as you use the ball, you will use your body for leverage in other exercises. You get a much broader range of motion with more muscles being engaged at once.

The exercises in Phase 2 are just plain fun! They become increasingly challenging with each phase, and by Phase 4, you will learn how to plan your own strength-training program using the exercises introduced in this book. Mentally, you'll have crossed over to the other side of the gym—and you won't even need to leave your living room!

The only piece of equipment you'll need for Phase 2 is the stability ball. You can buy one at many sports and discount stores, or you can order it from my Web site (www.chantelhobbs.com). I love using this tool because it's simple and portable and provides

Getting the Right Size

Stability balls come in different sizes. The right one for you depends on your height:

Up to 5'4"	45 cm ball
5'5"–5'7"	55 cm ball
5'8"–6'	65 cm ball
Over 6'	75 cm ball

an incredible workout. I've never felt better physically or experienced greater results from strength training than when I made the stability ball a permanent fixture in my workouts.

To design the strength-training program for this book, I consulted with my friend Joe Tedesco, a Duke-trained doctor of physical therapy and an all-around smart guy. I met Joe in a Spinning class I was teaching. I noticed this incredibly buff guy who took a bike in the front row and absolutely attacked it during class. If I said to do something, he did it with twice the intensity of anyone else in the room. I also noticed him doing some extensive stretches after class. I commented on them, and he explained that it was his profession and his passion. It was great to have Joe in class, because I knew I could pick his brain, and he'd give me helpful answers. Joe and his wife, Lesley, also a doctor of physical therapy, spoke to a group I was helping coach for a Disney Marathon. They covered injury prevention and the benefits of correct stretching. Not surprisingly, we were all impressed and learned a lot.

Joe was the perfect person to help me on my strength-training program. I value his knowledge and experience. He trains professional athletes, works with kids, rehabs people after injuries or surgery, and deals with elderly patients as well. He knows a lot about how the human body works. I tried to put all that knowledge into a strength-training program that will challenge you and make you much stronger and leaner than you've ever been, but at the same time it is 100 percent doable. Don't worry if some of the exercises seem difficult at first; they are designed to keep you wanting to do better. As you improve, each exercise has an option to challenge you further. As Joe and I both say regularly, rock on!

PHASE 2 EXERCISES

Do these ten exercises in one twenty-minute session. Do them twice a week, with at least one day in between to allow your muscles to recover and rebuild. Repetitions and sets of repetitions are listed for each exercise. Repetitions, known as reps, is the number of times to repeat each exercise to make a set. Do the number of sets listed, always resting between sets. If you find that the exercises are coming easily, and you'd like to push yourself harder, try the Challenge Yourself recommendation.

1. Bridge

This exercise challenges core stability, strengthening the spinal stabilizers, hamstrings, gluteal muscles, and calf muscles, and stretching the hip flexors. Attempting to minimize movement on the ball works the deep abdominal muscles and obliques.

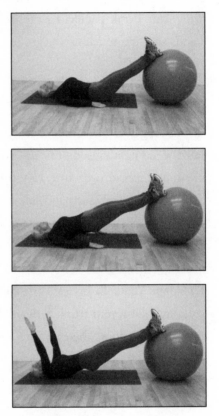

1. Begin with your back and arms flat on the floor and your heels resting on the ball.

2. Pushing against the floor with your hands and shoulders, lift your hips until your back and legs form a straight line, and hold momentarily. Return to the starting position, and repeat.

Challenge Yourself: Increase the difficulty by pointing your arms straight over your head and lifting your upper body by contracting your abdominal muscles.

	Week 5	Week 6	Week 7	Week 8
Reps	10	10	10	10
Sets	1–2	2	2–3	3

2. Trunk Lift with Arm T

This strengthens the middle- and lower-back muscles for improved posture, stabilizes the shoulder blades to prevent rounded shoulders, and stretches the chest muscles.

1. Lie on your stomach over the ball with your trunk parallel to the floor, hands and toes touching the ground.

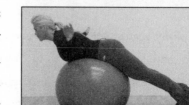

2. Keeping your head flat with eyes looking straight ahead, lift up your chest, and spread your arms to form a T, stopping when your hands are even with your shoulders. Return to the starting position, and repeat.

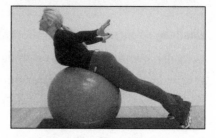

Challenge Yourself: Increase the difficulty by rolling your trunk forward on the ball while doing the exercise.

	Week 5	Week 6	Week 7	Week 8
Reps	10	10	10	10
Sets	1–2	2	2–3	3

3. Alternating Hip Extension

This strengthens the deep abdominal and lower-back muscles, strengthens glutes and hamstrings, stretches hip flexors, and trains the body to separate trunk and pelvis motions from hip and thigh motions to prevent lower-back injuries. The goal for this exercise is stability, not speed. Imagine balancing a glass of water on your lower back. Your mission: don't tip the glass over!

1. Lie on your stomach over the ball with your trunk parallel to the floor, hands and toes touching the ground.

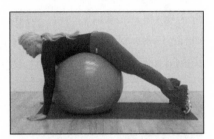

2. Lift one leg until it is parallel to the floor, keeping your back stationary. Return to the starting position, and repeat the exercise with the other leg.

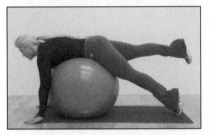

Challenge Yourself: Increase the level of difficulty by stretching one arm out while the opposite leg is being lifted.

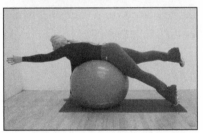

	Week 5	Week 6	Week 7	Week 8
Reps	10	10	10	10
Sets	1–2	2	2–3	3

4. Seated March

This strengthens sitting postural muscles to prevent neck and lower-back pain, tightens deep abdominal and lower-back muscles, improves sitting balance, incorporates ankles for balance training, and promotes stable, erect sitting posture.

1. Sitting erect on the ball with your shoulders down and back, your stomach drawn in, and your chest up, place your hands on the sides of the ball.

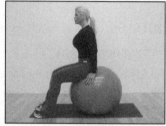

2. Keeping one knee bent, lift that foot off the floor, holding your starting posture throughout the lift. Repeat with the opposite leg to mimic a march.

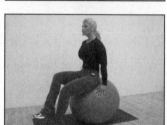

Challenge Yourself: Increase difficulty by lifting your arms from your sides while marching.

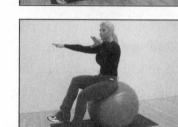

	Week 5	Week 6	Week 7	Week 8
Reps	10	10	10	10
Sets	1–2	2	2–3	3

5. Seated Abdominal Walk Out

By engaging the abdominals to resist falling backward, this exercise strengthens the abdominals while lengthening them, improving your balance and posture. It prepares the body for abdominal curls and improves total body coordination to create purposeful movement and proprioception (body awareness in space).

1. Sitting erect on the ball with your shoulders down and back, your stomach drawn in, and your chest up, place your hands on the sides of the ball.

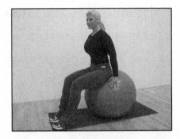

2. Slowly walk your feet out, using your thigh and stomach muscles, until your middle and lower back touches the ball. Tighten your stomach and thighs, and walk back up to the starting position.

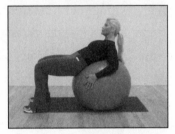

Challenge Yourself: Increase difficulty by walking your feet out until your shoulders and head are on top of the ball.

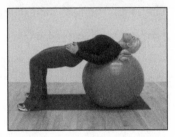

	Week 5	Week 6	Week 7	Week 8
Reps	10	10	10	10
Sets	1–2	2	2–3	3

6. Seated Diagonal Reaches

Keeping the trunk upright while moving several body parts at once improves the dynamic sitting posture. This incorporates obliques, spinal stabilizers, and shoulder-blade muscles to coordinate upper-body movement with lower-body stability and strengthen movements used in everyday life.

1. Sitting erect on the ball with your shoulders down and back, stomach drawn in, and chest up, place both hands on your Left thigh as close to the hip as possible.

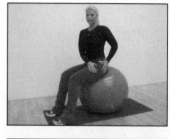

2. Reach both arms up diagonally to the Right, letting your head turn with the movement. Return to the starting position, and repeat. After ten repetitions, place both hands on your Right thigh and repeat the exercise, reaching to the Left.

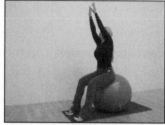

Challenge Yourself: Increase difficulty by performing the diagonal reach while also twisting from the waist in the same direction.

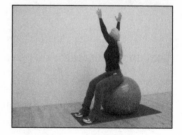

	Week 5	Week 6	Week 7	Week 8
Reps	10	10	10	10
Sets	1–2	2	2–3	3

7. Trunk Curl

This isolates the superficial abdominals during curling. The deep and oblique abdominals must also work to resist movement by stabilizing your body. The thigh and ankle muscles are engaged for balance and proprioception training.

1. Start with your shoulders and middle and lower back resting on the ball, your arms pointing straight up to the ceiling.

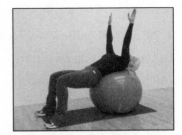

2. Curl your trunk up until your shoulders and upper back are off the ball, keeping your arms reaching away from your chest. Return to the starting position, and repeat.

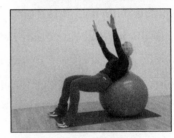

Challenge Yourself: Increase difficulty by curling an additional 45 degrees, until your arms are in front of you and aligned with your shoulders.

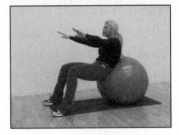

	Week 5	Week 6	Week 7	Week 8
Reps	10	10	10	10
Sets	1–2	2	2–3	3

8. Wall Squat

This incorporates thighs (quadriceps, hamstrings), gluteals, abdominals, and lower-back muscles for stabilization and erect posture, balancing with the ankles. It's a functional movement pattern that trains you to lift using the legs instead of rounding the back.

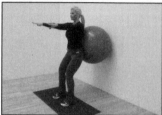

1. Stand with your lower back cupping the ball against a wall, arms reaching forward and ball just above your hips.

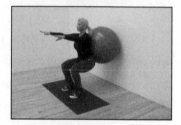

2. Lower your hips in a sitting motion by pushing into the ball, keeping your lower back against it. Roll downward, and stop when your knees are bent to no more than 90 degrees (a right angle). Roll upward, and return to the starting position, and repeat.

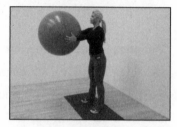

Challenge Yourself: Increase difficulty by holding the ball out in front of you and squatting until the ball taps the floor. Then return to standing upright.

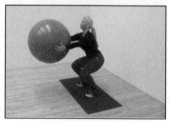

	Week 5	Week 6	Week 7	Week 8
Reps	10	10	10	10
Sets	1–2	2	2–3	3

9. Wall Lunge

This creates a narrow base of support to train lateral trunk stability. The glutes and thighs engage in a functional, forward-reaching motion to control the weight of the body, improving agility.

1. Stand holding the ball against a wall at arm's length and shoulder level.

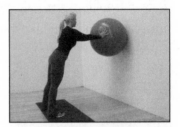

2. Using your arms to support your weight against the ball, step forward, bending one knee until your front thigh is parallel to the ground and you are in a lunge position. Do not let your front knee go beyond your toes. Step back to the starting position, and repeat with the other leg.

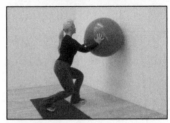

Challenge Yourself: Increase difficulty by holding the ball away from you—but not against a wall, so you are supporting the ball—and then stepping into the lunge position.

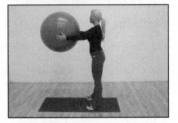

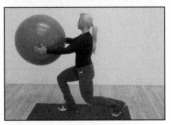

	Week 5	Week 6	Week 7	Week 8
Reps	10	10	10	10
Sets	1–2	2	2–3	3

10. Wall Push-up

This strengthens the chest, shoulders, and triceps and stabilizes the trunk by using abdominals to resist trunk extension, preventing lower-back problems.

1. Stand holding the ball against a wall at arm's length and shoulder level.

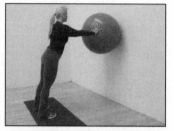

2. Lean into the ball by bending your arms to 90 degrees. Complete a push-up against the ball, returning to the starting position.

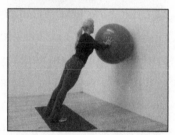

Challenge Yourself: Increase difficulty by performing the exercise on one foot by bending your knee and holding one foot off the ground.

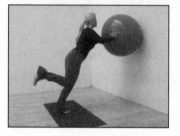

	Week 5	Week 6	Week 7	Week 8
Reps	10	10	10	10
Sets	1–2	2	2–3	3

Chapter 9

Phase 3 Make Food Boring

Weeks 9–12

Your Goal: to intensify your workouts and to break food's hold over you.

What You'll Need to Have
- Your new best friend—the stability ball
- Dumbbells
- A medicine ball, either 5 or 8 pounds

What You'll Need to Know
- What a 300-calorie meal looks like
- What protein, fat, and carbohydrates are and do

- How to choose food that produces maximum fuel
- Why interval training turbocharges your progress
- Why you add dumbbells and a medicine ball to your training
- How to choose your dumbbells

What You'll Need to Do

- Start the day with your Surrender Statement.
- Do cardio exercises four days per week, thirty minutes each day, and do one day with a twenty-minute interval session.
- Change up your cardio exercises to keep from getting bored.
- Do two days of strength training with thirty minutes each day with increased intensity.
- Begin to eat five small meals throughout the day, each being 200–400 calories, with a goal of 1,300–1,500 calories consumed each day.
- Create a personalized food list.
- Continue keeping your food journal.

If your idea of heaven is pondering all the great choices on the ten-page menu at A Certain Restaurant That Will Remain Nameless, then you are in for an eye-opening month. During Phase 3 you will change your eating habits so that food becomes *boring*. This will remove the power that food has over you and put it back in its proper place. Ready for a bombshell? Food shouldn't always be fun!

If this sounds like the worst news you've heard in a long time, remember you are now a very different person than you were when you started this program. You can do things you once believed were impossible. You have already made it through eight weeks. That's fifty-six days and nights that were anything but easy. You are living in a different way, thinking in a different way, and succeeding at things you never thought you'd do. In the process you've discovered how much self-control you have developed. Now, starting with Phase 3, you will discover that food doesn't have to be a major source of entertainment and pleasure. That's what family, friends, and Macy's are for!

We live in a world with far too many choices, and thinking about what to have for lunch or dinner becomes a major occupation for lots of people. I know; I was one of them. There is nothing wrong with thinking about enjoyable dinner plans. The problem is that the most unhealthy foods generally offer the best entertainment. Think about it: is it more fun to choose sundae toppings or salad toppings? No surprise that we end up in bondage to food, but even worse, we are also in bondage to the excitement that the endless choices give us. That's how food becomes a source of fun, a comforting friend, and even a therapist—to help you cope with the guilt of having repeatedly lost control over food.

I came to the painful realization that the only way for me to break such an emotional bond was to stop letting food control my thoughts. To do that, I had to rob food of its power by revealing it for what it truly is—fuel! Understanding this helped me remember the basic purpose of food: to keep me operating at an optimum level, thinking clearly, and feeling phenomenal.

> Rob food of its power by revealing it
> for what it truly is—fuel!

Gaining this perspective gave me the upper hand in my relationship with food. Once you start thinking of food this way, your decisions become much less complicated. Instead of asking yourself, *What am I in the mood for today?* you ask, *What does my body need?* Asking what you're in the mood for is one step away from making a poor choice. How often are you really in the mood for raw broccoli or spinach? Even when you manage to make the healthy choice, you can wear yourself out going through the mental gymnastics of deciding. Eliminate the whole ordeal this month, and you'll reduce your stress level and save a lot of time.

Many diets unintentionally make food choices more tantalizing by setting up a system of forbidden foods and reward foods. You get to look forward to a few especially exciting foods, but first you must save up your points. That can make you hyperaware of the foods you're craving, and that isn't what you want. Who needs more reasons to think about cheesecake? Instead, to gain power over food, you need to make the whole subject dull. Be willing to let food serve its higher and basic purpose of sustaining life—nothing more, nothing less.

"But wait!" you say. "Meals are the cornerstone of my family and social life. Food *has* to be one of my greatest pleasures in life!" I understand, and I want you to know that making food boring isn't a permanent life calling. Once you've broken food's spell and have learned to heed your body's desire for healthy Premium Fuel, you can start reintroducing a greater variety of foods into your life. In Phase 5 I will help you come to terms with your favorite foods again.

Staying in control long term is the key, and that's where most people fail. For now, you'll need to start thinking very differently about food, and you'll need to trust me. You may soon find that it's incredibly liberating to view food as simple fuel for your body and not a big social production. You may also be surprised at how much of your mental energy has gone into food decisions and find extra time and attention to devote to your workouts.

THE SAME SIMPLE LUNCH

I have a Type-AAA personality, so when I began to claim power over food, I went a little overboard. To make food boring, I ate the same lunch every day for months. It's what I needed to do to shrink food's prominence in my brain. There was a simple beauty to eating the same thing every day. It took no thought and created no stress in the middle of a hectic day—I just threw together my same turkey sandwich, and I was fueled up for the afternoon! If you really struggle to break bad food habits, you might want to try this. Eating the same healthy foods for months won't hurt you.

But some of you won't need to go quite this far. Instead, focus on eating five simple, healthy meals a day, using the list of foods later in this chapter as a guide. The goal is to learn what a 300-calorie meal looks like and eat one every few hours throughout the day. That way, food fantasies never have a chance to build uncontrollably. The meals won't be all that exciting, but they'll supply excellent fuel.

And they will taste good. I promise! With *Never Say Diet*, you get to plan your meals so you won't be stuck eating something you hate. I created a limited and basic list of things I knew would taste good to me, and those foods are what I ate regularly. It must have worked, because years later I still do the same thing. It was important that they be things I could stand to eat, or the whole exercise would have been pointless. If you try to force yourself to eat simple, healthy food that you hate, you'll never stick to it. Don't forget: this is *your* Brain Change and *your* new life. Learning to eat this way is one of the secrets of why you will never say diet again.

> ## Never-Say-Diet Tip
>
> Vagueness and variety are not your friends during Phase 3. Decide in advance when and what your workout will be each day. "I'll get to it eventually" basically means "Maybe I will, maybe I won't." That type of fuzziness means you're not telling yourself the truth.

When you design your list of foods, stay away from frozen diet entrées and processed foods; keep it natural. The point is to take control of your eating, not rely on others to make decisions and preportion things for you.

Eating 1,300 to 1,500 calories a day left me occasionally hungry, but that led to another important lesson. I learned to separate myself from the panic that usually accompanied hunger. Understanding metabolism helped me realize that being hungry didn't mean I automatically needed food. I had plenty of food stored up as fat, and that sensation of hunger meant that my body was switching over to the extra fuel tank—my fat stores.

LAUNCHING YOUR INTERVAL SESSIONS

Your body is changing all the time. Even when you can't see the changes, it is constantly adapting to what you force it to do. Old cells die, new cells get made, and sometimes they are very different cells. Over the course of a couple of years of workouts, you build an entirely new body! The more you push your body beyond its comfort zone, the faster it changes.

But you can push yourself only so far, right? It would be nice if you could rise off the couch and decide to start running five-minute miles, but it doesn't work that way. Within a few minutes of all-out running, you get exhausted. Further pushing can lead to injury or collapse.

Scientists, physiologists, and athletes have discovered that *interval training*—brief spurts of intense exercise, interspersed with gentler periods—delivers more benefits than moderately intense exercise alone. Why? Because the body has the chance to push really hard and then recover. A recent study found that most women, even nonathletic ones, were able to *double* their endurance after only a handful of interval sessions.[7]

The secret lies in the mitochondria, the tiny power plant in each of your cells. As we've discussed, mitochondria can burn either carbohydrates or fat, and they usually choose the carbs first. But when you push them hard, they have to switch over to fat. Push them hard regularly, and they begin burning the fat first and stay in fat-burning mode all the time, even during mild exercise and cool-down periods. In one major study, women burned 36 percent more fat during moderate cycling after a brief interval session than if they skipped the interval session and did just the lighter workout.[8]

It turns out that to trigger all the physiological changes you want—mitochondria switching over to burning fat, building new muscle, quickly increasing endurance—you don't have to push your body for long. Giving your body a taste of really hard work triggers all the same changes that a long, brutal workout does. With interval training, your body starts out even stronger the next time.

Now you understand why interval sessions will send your performance through the roof and rev up your resting metabolic rate as well. You accomplish more in a shorter period of time. But that doesn't mean you should do interval sessions all the time. As I said, part of the success of this training comes from giving your body time to rest. You should do interval sessions for short spurts, just one day a week during Phase 3 and two nonconsecutive days a week in Phase 4.

A Sample Interval Session

These days I do much of my interval training while Spinning, but you can do interval sessions with any cardio activity. Simply alternate periods of greater intensity with periods of recovery. Outdoor activities like walking or biking might naturally include intervals of hills that increase the difficulty, but, in general, indoor machines offer more control and information because you can see by the numbers in front of you how hard you are pushing. For example, on a treadmill you can increase the speed or incline, on an elliptical you can increase the strides or resistance, and on a stationary bike you can increase the resistance level or speed.

No matter how you do your interval sessions, you'll need to develop your own Perceived Exertion level, based on a scale of 1 to 10, where 2 is a gentle warmup, 4 is a normal steady pace, 6 is where you spend most of your cardio time, 8 is uncomfortable but doable, and at 10 you're considering dialing 911.

Your goal with interval sessions is to spend a good bit of time in the 6–10 area. Note that this Perceived Exertion scale is subjective and will change over time (as it should). A pace that feels like an uncomfortable 8 when you start may become an easy 4 after a few months.

If you wonder whether you are exercising hard enough, use the breath test. The majority of your cardio time should be spent at a steady heart rate (a 6 or 7 Perceived Exertion level), where you aren't gasping for breath but you can't carry on a long, constant conversation. A breath is needed in between sentences.

Because you build physical intensity more quickly through interval training, the best measure of your fitness is not how fast your heart rate gets with intense work efforts; it's how fast it comes back down afterward. That signals that your heart is ready to do it again! Consider getting a heart-rate monitor

Getting the Right Dumbbells

When it comes to buying dumbbells, you can go the route of purchasing individual sets, but I have found a more cost-effective way. First, if you are buying them individually, you should start with at least three sets. For most people, 5 pounds, 8 pounds, and 12 pounds work well. At my home gym I use an alternative called a Speed Pak. It's a universal set of dumbbells that can adjust from 3 to 15 pounds. Another set goes from 5 to 25 pounds. I believe this is the way to go because it is portable—I've been known to sneak it into the back of our Suburban for family road trips! Because they break down into five sets of varied weights, you get a lot for your money. You may already have dumbbells you want to add to, and that's fine. Both options are available on my Web site (www .chantelhobbs.com), at discount retailers such as Target, and at some sporting-goods stores.

and start paying attention to it during workouts and while at rest; you'll see the improvement as you become more fit. The time it takes to recover from intense exertion will become shorter with training and improved efficiency. I recommend a Polar heart-rate monitor—the simpler the better to start with. Extra buttons can lead to extra confusion.

Once you've established your Perceived Exertion scale, try the following routine for your interval session each week this month.

Minutes	Intensity
1–4	Gradually warm up to a steady pace (level 4), reaching level 5 by the fourth minute
5	Level 6
6	Level 7
7	Level 8
8	Level 9
9–10	Recover to level 4
11	Level 5
12	Level 6
13	Level 7
14	Level 8
15–16	Recover to level 5
17	Level 9
18	Level 10 for 30 seconds (you won't be able to stay there long) Level 6 for 30 seconds
19–20	Recover back to level 5

You should feel spent by the end of this interval, and you have spent extra calories! Be sure to take at least five additional minutes to cool down: levels 4, 3, 2, 1. Done!

THE THREE MUSKETEERS: PROTEIN, FAT, AND CARBS

You can be confident that you'll get solid, balanced nutrition by following the simple eating plan in *Never Say Diet*. The suggested menus, food combinations, and portion sizes have been checked and approved by Lon Ben-Asher, MS, RD. Lon holds degrees from the University of Florida and Florida International University. He serves as a clinical dietitian at North Shore Medical Center in Miami. Now it's time to talk about what you should eat.

All foods are made up of three types of nutrients, and unless you've been living on some other planet, you've heard plenty about them as one diet gets fashionable and another gets old. Low-fat diets, high-protein diets, low-carb diets—why would it make a difference what your food is made of? Because each type of nutrient serves a different function. Understanding what all three nutrients do will empower you in all your food decisions.

Protein is what animal muscle is made of. A steak is mostly protein. So is a salmon fillet. Turkey breast is almost pure protein. A few plant foods, such as beans and seeds, are high in protein, but most of our protein comes from animals. Protein builds new muscle and takes care of a host of higher functions within the body. Most of your body structure requires protein.

Protein, however, does not make good fuel. It doesn't burn easily or cleanly, so your body will only try to burn it if no carbohydrates or fats are available. It doesn't convert to fat easily either.

Carbohydrates—sugars and starches—are fuel. Energy. When a carrot grows thick and sweet with sugar, that's energy stored up for the plant (or us!). Grains are mostly carbohydrates. Picture a barn full of hay—that's a lot of stored energy, and it will burn hot and fast if you flick one match at it. Your body loves carbohydrates because they provide instant energy. Plant foods are mostly carbohydrates, whether in the form of a bowl of oatmeal or a Snickers Bar.

Fats are more like the timbers of the barn—much thicker and heavier than the straw. They'll burn too, but they usually need some help from the carbohydrates to get started. They store an amazing amount of energy, though, so once they start burning, they'll go all day.

A few calories of carbohydrates are stored right in your muscles, and when you instantaneously have to use your muscles for any reason, like catching a Frisbee coming at your head, these carbs get used first. After about a minute of activity, however, your muscles have used up their supplies, so more fuel comes rushing in through the blood. This fuel is carbohydrates stored in the blood and liver as glycogen—blood sugar. When you exercise, your insulin is responsible for pushing this energy out of your blood and into your muscles. That's why people who don't exercise can get high blood sugar and diabetes: they are pumping more sugar into their blood, but their muscles aren't sucking it out fast enough.

Exercise for more than twenty minutes, and you burn a lot of your carbohydrates. Your liver starts making more, but your body at this point switches over to its long-term energy system: fat. You have enough fat on your body to get you through a marathon and three more besides. Believe it or not, even skinny marathoners have enough fat for that. Burning fat requires *more* oxygen, which is why you start breathing harder as you exercise, especially on longer workouts.

Fat burns better when it's mixed with carbohydrates, and that's what your body does during long-term exertion, burning primarily fat with enough carbs mixed in to keep the fires burning bright. But if you exert yourself long and hard enough, you use up all your carbs, and your body has to get by on burning pure fat, which is a much slower energy-delivery process. This is where, when running a marathon, I have hit "the wall." For me, it usually happens around mile twenty.

Because fat is such a treasure-trove of energy, our bodies crave it. No news there! Fats (and oils, which are liquid fat) taste really good. They are essential to our health and even help us feel full. A little fat is a must in your diet, but because it is such a concentrated form of calories, it needs to be used in careful moderation. Part of the reason low-fat diets have a high likelihood of failure is because people never feel full, so they keep gobbling carbohydrates (pasta, potatoes, bread, rice), causing their blood sugar to spike and then crash.

Get Friendly with Fiber

Fiber isn't a nutrient like protein, fat, and carbohydrates, because your body can't digest fiber. In fact, that's the secret to fiber's benefit—it *can't* be digested. That's why it passes through the digestive system without contributing any calories. Better still, some types of fiber, called soluble fiber (the kind in oatmeal and bran), actually absorb fat and help prevent your body from ever digesting it, meaning fiber can cancel out some fat calories in your food.

Fiber is the tough stuff that holds plants together. You find it in the hard, outer wall of whole grains and the skin and interior of fruits, vegetables, and beans. You won't find any in animal products or in refined starches such as white flour or white rice, where it has been processed and stripped away. When people talk about complex carbohydrates versus simple ones, that's what they're talking about. A complex carb is a fruit, vegetable, or grain still in its natural form, mixed up with lots of fiber, which means your body has to work hard to break it down and extract the calories. Those calories trickle into your bloodstream much more slowly than the instant rush you get from simple carbs: white rice, white flour, potatoes, and sugar.

Eating lots of high-fiber foods will help you fill up on fewer calories, will slow the rate your body absorbs other calories, will reduce hunger, and will also aid in proper digestion and elimination. Fiber is an often-overlooked key to weight loss!

Your formula for healthy eating needs to be a mixture of protein, carbohydrates, and fat. Lots of protein to keep you lean and muscled, a little fat to make things taste good and to keep you full, and enough carbs to hold everything together while giving you some quick-burning fuel to keep your energy and metabolism high. The sample meals later in this chapter are designed to give you that nice, healthy mix.

YOUR FIVE-MEAL-A-DAY PLAN

Why do I recommend eating five small meals a day instead of the usual three large meals? Because the roller-coaster effect of three large meals, spaced hours apart, plays havoc with your blood sugar—and crashing blood sugar is a primary trigger of cravings and overeating. Space the same amount of calories over five meals, however, and your blood sugar never gets too high or too low. Grazing is the way to stay satisfied and lean. You will be able to better manage hunger pangs because your next meal is never more than a couple of hours away.

Keep in mind that this doesn't give you the freedom to eat five regular-sized meals a day. It's important to learn what a 300-calorie meal looks like and to eat about that many calories each meal. Notice that I don't recommend a shake for breakfast, a shake for lunch, and a sensible dinner. I want you to have real food at most meals, as well as an adequate amount of calories. Much less and you will put your body into starvation mode, which is a surefire way to lose control.

Since this is your own plan, it's perfectly fine to eat a 400-calorie meal at lunch if your midafternoon snack is only 200. Remember, one of the Five Decisions that you made is to be completely truthful with yourself, so if you exceed the combined-daily-calorie intake, the only person you are letting down is you. To lose weight, you must have a calorie deficit. Period.

The following are some examples of 300-calorie meals. They're listed by meal, but feel free to juggle them. It doesn't matter if you have the turkey wrap for breakfast and the veggie omelet for dinner. You can and should make your own substitutions to this list, or chuck it and create your own. But remember, the goal is to eat *boring* food this month. Variety may be the spice of life, but you have been overseasoning for too long. Easy, simple, and plain is better for now. Since you will be eating clean, choose your main staples right away and keep them available. ("Clean" is how I think about food that's simple, natural, and healthy and that keeps you energized.)

Don't stress out about precise calorie counts every meal. It's way too much work to try to weigh every morsel of food. In a short time of paying attention, you will develop a fairly close idea of where you stand. If in doubt, nutritional information is widely available on the Internet.

Creating Your Food List

Remember, don't say the D word! Instead, your task this month is to create a personalized list of sensible, healthy meals you will eat every week so you can *stop* paying attention to food. I know from talking to my clients that the main reason they tried so many other programs was the lure of the preplanning and calculating that had already been done for them. But if you never take ownership of your own nutrition (remember, that was one of your Five Decisions!), you won't achieve long-term change.

Here's what you do. Build your meals using the list of Premium Fuels provided later in this chapter. The list is not exclusive; feel free to substitute other proteins for the proteins listed here or other complex carbs for the carbs listed here, as long as your substitution isn't on the Bad Fuel list. Include a protein for at least four of your five daily meals, then fill in with carbs, vegetables, and the other Premium Fuels until you are in the 200-to-400-calorie range. Try to emphasize the veggies. Vegetables are vitamin-rich, complex carbohydrates and are mostly water, meaning they are low in calories. Nobody ever got fat eating veggies. (Plenty of people, however, get fat eating dressings, dips, butter, and cheese on their veggies—so watch out.) To get a feel for what a properly portioned minimeal looks like, check out my examples on the pages that follow, then substitute whatever similar-sized proteins and vegetables you want, or get a calorie counter and calculate your own.

Once you have created a week's worth of meals, eat the same meals for four weeks. Make it so regular that no mental energy goes into it. If you've followed the advice in this chapter, you'll know you're getting all the nutrients you need for high-level performance, and since food is fuel, that's all that matters.

I will warn you that if you have children, or a childlike husband, occasionally you will need to make something different for them to eat. But don't rule out kids' ability to like or try new foods, especially if you take the time to explain why this food is so good for them. My kids are a great example of this. I'm still amazed that all four of them enjoy salad, fish, and sweet potatoes.

Restaurant strategy: if you frequent a restaurant for lunch with your

Enjoy God's Candy Shop

It baffled my kids when I started eating clean. They were so used to riding in the grocery cart as I pushed it—slowly—down the cookie aisle. Suddenly I had to speed past the cookies, look the other way, and head straight to produce. One day I was trying to explain to my daughter Kayla, who was four years old and my mini-me, why we needed to skip the free sugar cookie from the bakery and buy apples instead. I said, "Honey, this apple is made by God. It's the very best candy you can buy." She looked confused and said, "Didn't He make M&M's for that?" I laughed. But we kept hanging out at the produce department, and now Kayla is eleven and loves fruits and vegetables. I know that once you get hooked on them, you'll think they are God's candy too!

co-workers or dinner with family or friends, make sure your food list for the month includes something you can find on the menu. For instance, I can always order a chicken sandwich and take off the top slice of bread or order salads—dressing always on the side. There are very few places, including fast-food restaurants, where you can't find something acceptable.

When it comes to protein bars, let me say this: they are convenient, and there is a place for that. But try to limit them. They are highly processed and are often high in saturated fat as well as sugar. I think Kashi makes a great nutrition bar: the calories are low, the fiber is high, and the taste is great.

I also drink protein shakes. To make one, I use a protein powder that is low in sugar, and I add skim milk and some frozen fruit. They work well for my busy life, and I never get tired of drinking them. They give me energy and satisfy the need for a significant amount of protein at once, especially after an intense strength-training session when it can aid in muscle repair.

Some of my recommended foods contain sugar substitutes, which can be valuable tools for cutting calories. Many people, however, aren't comfortable eating the artificial ingredients. I support the desire to eat all-natural foods; just remember that your daily calorie goal remains the same.

THE PREMIUM FUEL LIST

Protein

Extra-lean ground beef	Eggs
Lean ground sirloin	Egg whites
Chicken breast	Egg Beaters
Turkey breast	Trout
Lean ground turkey	Scallops
Lean ham	Snapper
Lean pork loin	Cod
Extra-lean turkey bacon	Halibut

Protein *(continued)*

Swordfish

Haddock

Salmon

Crab

Shrimp

Water-packed tuna

Low-fat cottage cheese

Veggie burgers

Tofu

Carbohydrates—Complex

Sweet potatoes

Yams

Squash

Corn

Rice (brown or wild)

Pasta (whole-wheat)

Oatmeal

Whole-wheat bread

Whole-wheat crackers

Whole-wheat tortillas

High-fiber cereals

Beans, Legumes, Seeds, and Nuts

Black beans

Garbanzo beans (chickpeas)

Kidney beans

Lentils

Lima beans

Navy beans

Pinto beans

Soybeans

Miso

Almonds

Cashews

Peanuts

Pecans

Walnuts

Flax seeds

Pumpkin seeds

Sunflower seeds

Fruits

Apples

Apricots

Bananas

Blueberries

Cantaloupe

Cranberries

Fruits (continued)

Figs

Grapefruit

Grapes

Kiwis

Lemons

Limes

Oranges

Papayas

Pears

Pineapples

Plums

Prunes

Raisins

Raspberries

Strawberries

Watermelon

Vegetables

Artichokes

Asparagus

Beets

Bell peppers

Broccoli

Brussels sprouts

Cabbage

Carrots

Cauliflower

Celery

Collard greens

Cucumbers

Eggplant

Fennel

Garlic

Green beans

Green peas

Kale

Leeks

Lettuce

Mushrooms

Mustard greens

Olives

Onions

Parsley

Spinach

Tomatoes

Zucchini

ALTERNATIVE FUELS

These foods may be necessary to complete meals or snacks. Some are high in calories, however, so use in moderation.

Low-fat/fat-free cheese

Low-fat/fat-free sour cream

Milk—1 percent or skim

Fat-free yogurt

Baked potatoes

Peanut butter (natural is best)

Almond butter

Low-fat cream cheese

Fruit spreads

Mustard

Avocados

Hummus

Salsa

Juice—low-sugar

Ketchup

Light mayonnaise

Snack Ideas

Here are some snack ideas that I call the six Ps. I like them because they cover all the taste cravings—cold, sweet, crunchy, and salty. Limit consumption of these to one a day.

Pudding (fat free)

Popsicles (sugar free)

Popcorn (plain or fat free)

Pretzels (fat free, unsalted)

Pickles (low sodium)

Protein bar (less than three grams of saturated fat)

Use Sparingly—Oils, Sauces, Dressings, and Marinades

Olive oil

Safflower oil

Canola oil

Sunflower oil

Flaxseed oil

Low-sodium soy sauce

Artificial sweeteners

Low-fat/light salad dressings

THE BAD-FUEL LIST

All sweets and salty snacks

Chips

Processed snacks—cereal bars, Pop-Tarts, waffles, etc.

White bread and white flour

Sugar and honey

Fatty meats (steak, pork, bacon, sausage, etc.)

Butter and cream

Full-fat cheese and milk

High-calorie drinks (juices, soft drinks, sweetened tea and coffee,
   alcohol)

EXAMPLES OF RIGHT-PORTIONED MEALS

Counting calories is about as exciting as sorting socks, but being able to eye-ball a meal and have a general sense of its caloric content is an essential aspect of your long-term weight maintenance. Use these sample meals for ideas and as guidelines. Once you've been eating them for a while, you'll be able to substitute other foods from the same nutrition categories and have a good guesstimate of the calories. Try to stick to what you know.

For example, I knew the exact calorie content of this sandwich:

My Infamous Turkey Sandwich

2 slices of Nature's Own bread (fiber rich, whole grain)
   = 100 calories

6 slices of turkey (pure protein) = 100 calories

1 dab of mayo (to make it stick) = 25 calories

2 pickles (a little salty) = 50 calories

Lettuce, onion, and tomato (for crunch and flavor) = 25 calories

Total: 300 calories

To get you started, here are a number of other meals that all fall around that 300-calorie total, with the three main meals being a little higher and the two snack meals being a little lower.

Meal #1—Five Breakfast Options (300–400 Calories)

- Oatmeal, 2 tablespoons raisins, 3 slices turkey bacon
- Veggie egg white / Egg Beater omelet (chopped green pepper, onion, tomato), 1 tablespoon fat-free cheese, 1 banana
- Slice of whole-grain toast, 1 tablespoon peanut butter, 1 cup Kashi GoLean cereal, 1 cup skim milk
- 1/2 whole-grain English muffin, 1 tablespoon all-fruit jam, scrambled Egg Beaters, 3 slices turkey bacon
- Protein shake with 1 cup skim milk, 1 cup strawberries, 1/2 banana

Meal #2—Five Options for a Midmorning Snack (200–300 Calories)

- 1 cup Dannon Light 'n Fit yogurt, 2 tablespoons low-fat granola, 1 cup frozen blueberries
- 5 deli slices of turkey breast (4 ounces), 1 pear, 10 whole cashews
- 2 rice cakes, 2 tablespoons almond butter, 1 orange
- Protein shake with 1 cup skim milk and 1/2 banana
- 5 deli slices of chicken breast, 1 apple, 10 whole pecans

Meal #3—Five Lunch Options (300–400 Calories)

- Salad, grilled chicken, 2 tablespoons light balsamic dressing, 2 tablespoons hummus, 1/2 whole-wheat pita
- Turkey wrap: 4 ounces sliced turkey breast, whole-wheat tortilla, dab of light mayo, lettuce, onion, tomato, 1 orange
- 4 ounces tuna with 2 tablespoons light mayo on bed of romaine lettuce, 2 tablespoons almond slices, 1 orange
- 4 ounces chopped chicken, 3/4 cup brown rice, 3/4 cup black beans, 3 tablespoons salsa
- Grilled chicken breast, 1 tablespoon barbecue sauce, broccoli, low-fat granola bar

Meal #4—Five Afternoon-Snack Options (200–300 Calories)

- Kashi GoLean Bar, 1 cup cantaloupe
- 1 cup carrots, $1/2$ cucumber, 2 tablespoons light ranch dressing, 20 whole almonds
- 15 frozen grapes, 4 slices turkey breast
- $1/4$ cup cranraisins, $1/4$ cup Kashi GoLean cereal, 1 cup Dannon Light 'n Fit yogurt
- 2 cups popcorn, 1 Granny Smith apple

Meal #5—Five Options for Dinner (300–400 Calories)

- Herb-baked salmon, $3/4$ cup brown rice, sautéed spinach with chopped garlic and olive oil
- Teriyaki-grilled chicken breast, $1/2$ sweet potato with cinnamon, salad, 2 tablespoons light dressing
- 6 ounces Shake 'n Bake lean pork loin, steamed veggies, $3/4$ cup couscous
- 2 lean sirloin fajitas (6 ounces), green peppers, onions, 4 tablespoons salsa, 2 tablespoons fat-free cheese, 2 tablespoons fat-free sour cream
- 6 ounces roasted turkey breast, small potato, spinach salad with 2 tablespoons light dressing

PHASE 3 EXERCISES

Do the following ten exercises in one thirty-minute session. Do them twice a week, with at least one day in between to allow your muscles to recover and rebuild. Reps and sets are listed for each one. "Reps" is the number of times you repeat each exercise to make a set. Do the number of sets listed, always resting between sets. Each exercise includes a Challenge Yourself recommendation, which you can use if you find the exercises are coming easily and you'd like to push yourself harder. Most of these exercises use a stability ball.

1. Bridge with Hamstring Curl

This strengthens the lower back and improves gluteal and hamstring strength.

1. Lie flat on your back with your arms on the floor alongside your body, heels and calves resting on the stability ball, and your legs straight. Draw your abdomen in and squeeze your glutes and the backs of your thighs to raise your buttocks four to six inches off the floor.

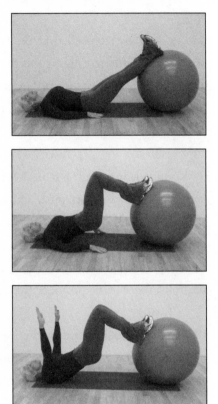

2. While your buttocks are in the air, bend your knees by digging your heels into the ball. Slowly straighten your legs and return to the starting position and repeat.

Challenge Yourself: Perform the exercise with your arms held straight up in the air to decrease stability and increase your core muscle activation.

	Week 9	Week 10	Week 11	Week 12
Reps	10	10	10	10
Sets	1–2	2	2–3	3

2. Back Extension with Shoulder Blade W Squeezes

This strengthens the upper-back postural muscles—to prevent rounded shoulders—and tightens the hamstring and gluteals.

1. Lie on your stomach over the ball with your hands resting on the floor. Draw your abdomen in and squeeze your glutes as you raise your chest up off the ball.

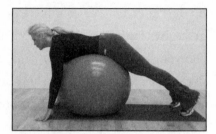

2. Keeping your head and neck in a straight line with your spine, squeeze your shoulder blades together and raise your arms out to the sides to form a W. Slowly lower your chest and arms to return to the starting position. Repeat.

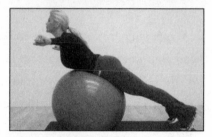

Challenge Yourself: Perform the exercise with a medicine ball in your hands, pulling it to your chest as you squeeze together your shoulder blades.

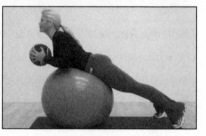

	Week 9	Week 10	Week 11	Week 12
Reps	10	10	10	10
Sets	1–2	2	2–3	3

3. Side-Lying Leg Raises

This strengthens the lateral hips and improves lateral trunk stability by recruiting the obliques.

1. Lie on your Right side over the ball, your ribs, waist, and hip against the ball, and your Right hand touching the floor. Use your Left hand to stabilize the ball. Stack your feet on top of each other with your legs held straight and together and with your Right foot resting on the floor.

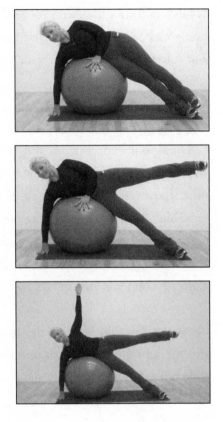

2. Draw your abdomen in and lift your Left leg until it is parallel with the ground. Stabilize your body by tightening your abdominal muscles. Slowly lower your leg to the starting position and repeat. After ten repetitions, switch your body to the Left side and repeat the lift using your Right leg.

Challenge Yourself: Perform the exercise with one arm extended overhead in a straight line with your other arm touching the ground.

	Week 9	Week 10	Week 11	Week 12
Reps	10	10	10	10
Sets	1–2	2	2–3	3

4. Alternating Arm and Leg Raises

This improves lower-back stability by separating trunk and pelvic stabilization from hip motion.

1. Lie flat on your back with your arms over your head on the floor, your heels and calves on the ball with your legs straight.

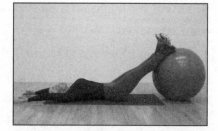

2. Draw your abdomen in, and raise your Right arm and Left leg at the same time. Touch your Right hand to your Left shin. Return to the starting position, and raise your Left arm and Right Leg, touching the shin. Continue alternating the opposite arm and leg.

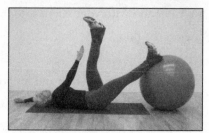

Challenge Yourself: Perform the exercise by reaching for your ankle using an abdominal curl-up.

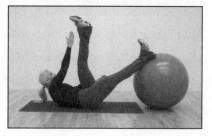

	Week 9	Week 10	Week 11	Week 12
Reps	10	10	10	10
Sets	1–2	2	2–3	3

5. Push-up

This incorporates abdominals, lower-back muscles, gluteals, and hamstrings to stabilize the trunk, while strengthening chest, triceps, and shoulder stabilizers.

1. Lie on your stomach over the ball with your hands on the floor and your arms shoulder width apart, pelvis on top of the ball, and feet off the floor. Keep your knees straight.

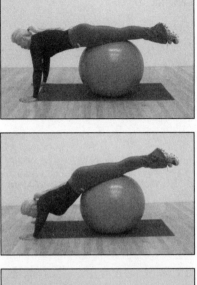

2. Draw in your abdomen, and slowly lower your chest by bending your elbows to 90 degrees. Straighten your elbows by pushing your palms into the floor, and raise up to the starting position, and repeat.

Challenge Yourself: Perform the exercise with your knees or shins (instead of your pelvis) on top of the ball.

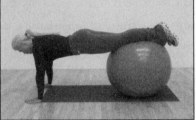

	Week 9	Week 10	Week 11	Week 12
Reps	10	10	10	10
Sets	1–2	2	2–3	3

6. Dumbbell Triceps Extension

This incorporates abdominals, lower-back muscles, gluteals, and hamstrings to stabilize the trunk, and strengthens the triceps. For the last two reps, choose a dumbbell weight that challenges you but isn't so heavy that it causes you to sacrifice form.

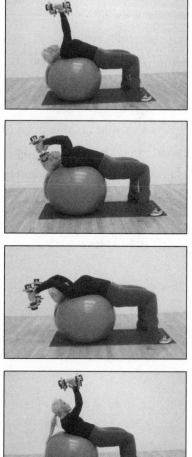

1. Lie on your back over the ball with your outstretched arms holding dumbbells straight up, shoulders on top of the ball and feet flat on the floor and shoulder width apart.

2. Keeping your elbows over your shoulders, slowly lower the dumbbells toward your head by bending your elbows to 90 degrees. Stop when the dumbbells are in line with your forehead. Straighten your arms to return to the starting position with wrists, elbows, and shoulders aligned.

Challenge Yourself: Perform the exercise starting with your arms outstretched past your head. Crunch with your abdominals while you pull the dumbbells up and forward, keeping your arms as straight as possible.

	Week 9	Week 10	Week 11	Week 12
Reps	10	10	10	10
Sets	1–2	2	2–3	3

7. Bent-over Dumbbell Row

This incorporates trunk stability by challenging the lower-back muscles, gluteals, and thighs; strengthens shoulder blades and upper-back muscles; and incorporates ankle stability for balance.

1. Bend forward into lunge position with your trunk parallel to the floor and your outstretched Right hand on the ball for support. Your Left arm should be dropped at your side holding a dumbbell.

2. Draw in your abdomen, and slowly squeeze your Left shoulder blade as you bend your Left elbow while pulling up the dumbbell. Keep pulling up the dumbbell until your Left elbow bends to 90 degrees. Keep the elbow close to your side. Slowly lower the weight to the starting position, and repeat with the other arm.

Challenge Yourself: Perform the exercise while bending your knee 90 degrees and holding one foot off the floor (the foot on the side opposite the arm lifting the weight).

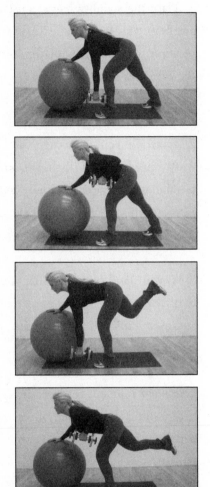

	Week 9	Week 10	Week 11	Week 12
Reps	10	10	10	10
Sets	1–2	2	2–3	3

8. Squat with Hammer Press

This incorporates the entire body (lower back, abdominals, gluteals, thighs, arms, and shoulders) to functionally improve total body power.

1. Place the stability ball against a wall and lean your back against it in a squat position, your lower back supported by the ball. Your arms should be dropped at your sides, holding dumbbells.

2. Draw in your abdomen, and push with your glutes and thighs as you begin to stand up. At the same time, bend your elbows and curl the dumbbells up to shoulder level.

3. As you stand up higher, use your legs to drive the dumbbells in one motion up and over your head. Slowly return to the starting position, and repeat.

Challenge Yourself: Perform the exercise in one fluid motion without using the ball for support.

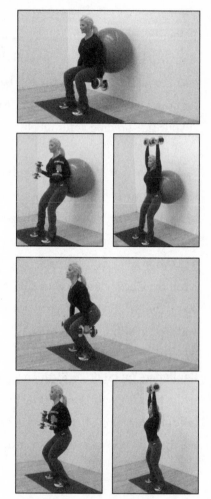

	Week 9	Week 10	Week 11	Week 12
Reps	10	10	10	10
Sets	1–2	2	2–3	3

9. Diagonal Reach-ups

This incorporates the entire body (lower back, abdominals, gluteals, thighs, arms, and shoulders) to functionally improve total body power in multiple planes.

1. Stand with your feet slightly wider apart than your shoulders, knees bent slightly, and hands above your Right knee.

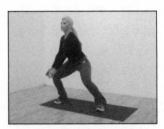

2. Push with your thighs as you stand up and lift. Let your head follow your hands as you twist your trunk to the Left and reach up to the ceiling with your hands. Pull back to the starting position, hands above your Right knee, as fast as you can by squeezing your abdominal muscles. Repeat with the other side.

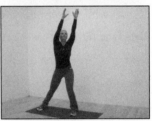

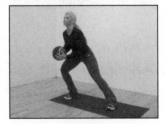

Challenge Yourself: Perform the exercise while holding a medicine ball, or increase speed without sacrificing technique.

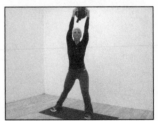

	Week 9	Week 10	Week 11	Week 12
Reps	10	10	10	10
Sets	1–2	2	2–3	3

10. Side Lunge with Reach

This incorporates the entire body (lower back, abdominals, gluteals, thighs, arms, and shoulders) to functionally improve lateral body movement.

1. Stand upright with your hands dropped at your sides and your feet shoulder width apart.

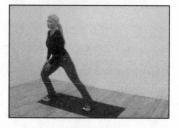

2. Draw in your abdomen, and step to the Right while keeping your trunk upright. Reach your hands to your Right knee, and shift your weight to the Right thigh by bending your Right knee. Return to the starting position, and repeat. After ten repetitions do the same exercise, going to the Left.

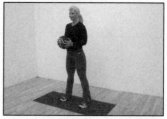

Challenge Yourself: Perform the exercise while holding a medicine ball.

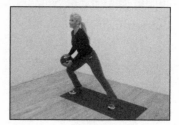

	Week 9	Week 10	Week 11	Week 12
Reps	10	10	10	10
Sets	1–2	2	2–3	3

Chapter 10

Phase 4
Get Strong

Weeks 13–16

Your Goal:
to intensify your workouts while beginning to reward yourself for your progress.

What You'll Need to Have

- Your new best friend—the stability ball
- Dumbbells
- A medicine ball
- Clothes to sweat in
- A plastic tape measure

What You'll Need to Do

- Start the day with your Surrender Statement.

- For cardio, do four days of thirty minutes and one day of a twenty-minute interval session.
- Do three days of strength training for thirty minutes with added intensity.
- Keep eating clean, but test and reward yourself with one indulgent meal each week.
- Weigh yourself weekly.
- Continue taking your measurements.
- Continue keeping your food journal.

The theme for Phase 4 is your strength, both inside and out! You are going to make yourself physically stronger than you've ever been through some pretty intense strength training. At the same time, you will test your mental toughness with one indulgent meal every week during Phase 4. Why push it? Because when all is said and done, you're going to end this month with incredible confidence. You'll be someone who knows that no force on earth could knock you off your path.

When I entered this phase, in every way I was feeling stronger than I ever had before. I had become good at resisting temptation, and I was meeting new fitness goals all the time. I was also hearing lots of compliments, which made me want to keep it up! I had to get rid of clothes that were too big and replace them with smaller sizes, which was a lot more fun than doing it the other way around! I also felt closer to God than I could ever remember. I had come to depend on Him each day to keep me strong and focused. It was a very exciting time in my life, and I felt I was ready for anything.

But I'd be lying if I said I didn't occasionally miss some of my favorite foods. Eventually I wanted to have the flexibility to eat a delicious meal with friends or my husband and not have it send me into a downward spiral. But weight loss was still my top priority, and I had a long way to go. My goal was eventually to live with an 80/20 mentality: Eat clean Premium Fuels 80 percent of the time; allow myself Regular Fuels 20 percent of the time. As long as I kept exercising, I figured I could maintain my weight without dieting or missing out on too many good times.

Any journey is easier if there are incentives and rewards along the way. For me to be able to do this for the long haul, I needed something to look forward to occasionally, or I'd become a burned-out statistic. People don't plan to go off their diets; they falter when the mental pressure gets too intense. I had a strategy to prevent this: I would set a time in advance when I would allow myself an indulgence. Then I wouldn't start feeling deprived or sorry for myself, and I'd be able to resist temptation the rest of the time. Here's how I set it up: one meal, once a week, no holds barred!

I started planning that first meal days ahead of time. It would be a Friday-night date for Keith and me, and it would be the perfect meal. I had Outback Steakhouse's Chocolate Thunder From Down Under ordered in my head three days in advance. We arrived and started with some cheese fries. Cheese fries! After a month of turkey breast, they were ridiculously yummy. Yet I couldn't help pointing out to Keith how many calories were in the ranch dipping sauce. He smiled and asked me please not to ruin his dinner. "But, baby, I can't help it," I replied. "It's what I do now." He said, "How about you do it in your head, not out loud?" How times had changed!

I had a salad next—something wholesome—and I didn't dare touch the bread. I wanted to maintain some control. Next came my perfectly cooked steak and loaded baked potato. I tried to forget about the calories and the high fat content in the big slab of beef and the enormous potato covered with butter, sour cream, cheese, and bacon. I reminded myself that I didn't do this every day, and I cut into that steak like it was my last meal. It was sensational.

But that was just a warmup to the main event, what my husband refers to as "sex on a plate"—the Chocolate Thunder From Down Under. It arrived— a warm brownie smothered in hot fudge and topped with vanilla ice cream and fresh whipped cream. By then I was eating way past hunger, way past full, and well into "I think I might be sick." I hadn't been there in a long time.

And you know what? It wasn't fun. Not even a little bit entertaining. Then a pretty crazy thing happened. Several bites into my dream dessert, after two months of deprivation and days of anticipation, I put my spoon down and went home. I felt bloated, sick, and irritated. I couldn't believe I'd once been a person who used to push myself to eat that much on a regular basis. My body didn't want that much food, and my brain knew better even as the spoon was going in. Had I changed more than I realized?

All week I'd been thinking about that dessert…and it looked just as good

Never-Say-Diet Tip

No matter how much I tell people they should weigh in only once a week, I know that many of them weigh themselves more frequently. This is entirely your choice. Just try not to put too much emphasis on any one day's reading. Everyone's weight fluctuates, mostly because we are nearly 70 percent water. And for those of us who exercise, tearing down muscle means rebuilding it as well. This requires extra fluid, which can mean retaining more water. For all these reasons, your weight loss will not be a perfectly smooth downward line. It may go up a few pounds and then down a few, and then down again and up one. All that matters is the downward trend over a month's time. Don't let the number on the scale control your mood for the day.

as I'd imagined. But I didn't enjoy it as much as I'd expected. As each bite of dessert had gone into my mouth, thoughts had come flooding in: *Great, here you go again! Wow, on just one meal you blew several days of working out!*

Was I a failure? a cheat? I worried that I still had serious food issues I'd never be able to move beyond. I felt guilty, sick, and angry with myself. This was not in the plan. All I could do that night was pray. Surrendering is my insurance. I asked God to keep me strong and help me deal with my feelings. No one could understand how I was feeling; this was old guilt from my past.

I went to sleep, woke up the next day, and, yes, the scale had moved 3 pounds—in the wrong direction. *Relax,* I told myself. *I couldn't have gained 3 pounds from just one meal.* (Much later I'd learn how our body processes food and why the extra sugar and salt caused this big fluctuation.)

At the time I was so concerned and aggravated that I thought about skipping breakfast. No, that would just make me hungrier later. Then I thought about doing an extra hour of cardio to punish myself. Finally I got a grip. This was not a race. I didn't need to redouble the speed of my progress, because there was no finish line! Since I wasn't on a diet, I couldn't have cheated; therefore I didn't need to be punished.

The next few days I simply went about doing my new job—eating Premium Fuels and working out on schedule—and I moved on. By the time I weighed myself the following week, my weight was back down, and I had lost another 2 pounds. Good news! I hadn't blown it; I was in control, and I was never the same from then on.

It took many more "free" meals for me to be able to relax and enjoy them. But I have found that as long as I don't stuff myself, as long as I slow down and stop eating while I still feel good, there is no guilt, just satisfaction.

I felt stronger by the end of Phase 4 because I had tasted freedom and recognized that I had the power not to abuse it. Food no longer controlled me; I controlled it. A huge peak moment!

Learn to Crave Premium Fuel

And that's why I suspect the latest round of diet experts may be clueless. They like to tell us that overeating is genetic, that even if you lose a lot of weight, you will inevitably develop an uncontrollable need to pack it back on, or your addictive personality may turn to drugs or alcohol to replace overeating. Well, I'm sorry, but those theories don't describe my experience. Once I started to lose weight and got a taste of what being healthy and eating sensibly was like, I couldn't stand to stuff myself. I'd had a number of peak moments over the previous months, and I was living a new life. Overeating felt bad. It could never compete with the great feeling of eating clean, exercising, and getting fit.

Your brain really can change—and your body with it. I'm living proof. As you put a substantial amount of time into living better than you ever have before, you want to feel that way permanently and will do whatever it takes. Somehow the diet police haven't figured this out yet. Maybe enough of us need to prove them wrong!

That's where my program parts ways with so many of the diets out there. At one time getting to eat a diet brownie every day sounded good, as did prepackaged entrées and the lure of a magic, fat-burning, thermogenetic pill. But none of these approaches can offer long-term success. They just cause you to stay trapped in dieting cycles, where you make temporary progress, then lose ground, and then once again try to get your head back in the game. They don't tell you that the only way to permanent freedom is to make your body crave premium stuff most of the time and to rerig your mind to commit to the value of going without. I understand why. That message isn't as catchy as "Have your dessert every day, and lose weight too!" but we need to hear it. Remember, *Never Say Diet* is based on telling ourselves the truth.

When you develop a strong exercise habit, as you have done, and you understand the power that it has on what you eat, then your body, your machine, starts to beg for the best fuel you can give it. By desiring the best, it also rejects the low-quality stuff. Ever put cheap gas in your car after it has been running on high test? It doesn't run as smoothly as before. This happens in your body too. And it helps your mind to make the connection between feeling good and eating good. They go together.

Here in Phase 4 this will really kick in. And that's why it's time to test yourself with some planned freedom. When you first got on this bike, it had training wheels because, like me, you needed them. You had fallen off many times before and were frustrated. But now it's time to remove the training wheels for just a few minutes and to practice riding on your own! Not completely—that will come in Phase 5. For now, give yourself one celebration meal each week. Let it be whatever you want. Be sure to look forward to it during the difficult workouts! I want you to completely enjoy it. But don't feel like you have to eat like you used to. You know yourself so much better now, and you may be surprised by what you choose as your celebration meal.

> *When you develop a strong exercise habit, your body starts to beg for the best fuel you can give it.*

THE REWARDS OF PHASE 4

This month will be extremely rewarding. You are becoming so efficient at burning fat and building muscle that you will start to see significant changes in your body.

I get superexcited about the strength training in Phase 4. Continue doing three nonconsecutive days for thirty minutes each day. However, for one of those three sessions, design your own workout. This is where you get to take charge and *own* your fitness plan! That will make all the difference once you have completed the sixteen weeks of the Brain Change.

I once heard a child-rearing expert say, "Why would you hand your kids money as they need it while they live at home, without much instruction, and then send them out into the world with their own checkbook and credit card and expect them not to bounce a check or max out their credit?" For any of us to really get things right and make the best decisions, we need to learn and practice a little at a time, especially when our lifelong success is on the line. For your three strength-training sessions each week, use the exercises described here in Phase 4 for one session and then the exercises from Phase 3 for the next session (that will give you a full-body workout). And for the third session, choose any ten exercises from the thirty in Phases 2–4, including the Challenge Yourself options. This is an opportunity for you to decide which exercises you like, which ones are easy, and which ones make you work a little harder. It's up to you to determine the level of intensity.

You'll need to write down your strength-training plan. Make copies of the following pages so you can not only record the exercises but also make notes on how things are going with each one. (You can also download these pages from my Web site: www.chantelhobbs.com.) Write the names of the ten exercises you choose, as well as the number of reps you plan for each. Use the notes section to record information, such as whether you were able to do the exercise as you planned, how it felt, whether you could improve, and what to change, depending on how you did. If it was easy, list ways you can make it more difficult, and if it was too much and you had trouble completing it correctly, come up with ways to make it more doable. Refer back to these notes the next time you do the workout so you'll keep improving.

Have fun; you're ready to grab the handlebars and take off!

Your Strength-Training Plan

DATE: _____
EXERCISE 1 _____   REPS _____
NOTES _____
_____
_____

DATE: _____
EXERCISE 2 _____   REPS _____
NOTES _____
_____
_____

DATE: _____
EXERCISE 3 _____   REPS _____
NOTES _____
_____
_____

DATE: _____
EXERCISE 4 _____   REPS _____
NOTES _____
_____
_____

DATE: _____
EXERCISE 5 _____   REPS _____
NOTES _____
_____
_____

DATE:_____
EXERCISE 6 _____   REPS _____
NOTES _____
_____
_____

DATE:_____
EXERCISE 7 _____   REPS _____
NOTES _____
_____
_____

DATE:_____
EXERCISE 8 _____   REPS _____
NOTES _____
_____
_____

DATE:_____
EXERCISE 9 _____   REPS _____
NOTES _____
_____
_____

DATE:_____
EXERCISE 10 _____   REPS _____
NOTES _____
_____
_____

Phase 4 Exercises

Do the following ten exercises in one of your three thirty-minute sessions each week. Allow at least one day in between sessions for your muscles to recover and rebuild. Reps and sets are listed for each. Do the number of sets listed, always resting between sets. Remember to use the Challenge Yourself recommendations if you find that the exercises are coming easily and you'd like to push yourself harder.

1. Bridge with Alternate Leg Lift

This strengthens the lower-back stabilizers and improves eccentric gluteal and hamstring strength.

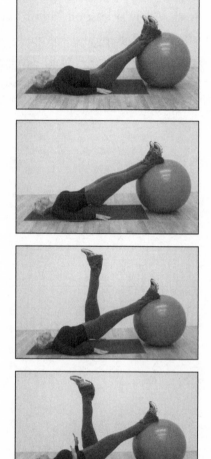

1. Lie flat on your back with your hands and arms on the floor at your sides, palms down on the ground, and your buttocks resting on the floor. Rest your heels and calves on the stability ball with your legs straight. Draw in your abdomen, squeeze the back of your thighs, and raise your buttocks four to six inches off the floor.

2. Reinforce your glutes and back-of-thigh contraction, and raise your Right leg off the ball until it's nearly vertical. Keeping your body still, slowly lower your leg to the ball, keeping your buttocks in the air. Repeat with your Left leg, and continue to alternate.

Challenge Yourself: Perform the exercise with your arms bent so that your elbows support you, rather than your palms and elbows, with just your upper torso on the floor, to decrease stability and increase core-muscle activation.

	Week 13	Week 14	Week 15	Week 16
Reps	10	10	10	10
Sets	1–2	2	2–3	3

2. Core Planks

This incorporates abdominal and lower-back stabilization and uses hip flexor and thigh muscle activation to resist trunk extension and challenge core stability.

1. Kneel on the floor with the stability ball in front of you. Place your bent elbows on top of the ball, toes bent and pushing against the floor.

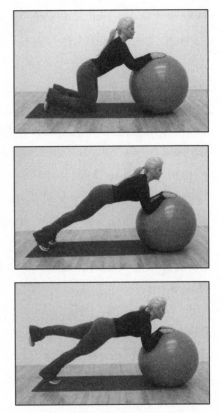

2. Draw in your abdomen, squeeze the front and back of your thighs, and raise your knees off the floor. Lift until your legs are straight, creating a long straight line from head to toe. Reinforce the abdominal contraction as you shift your weight to balance your body using elbows, shoulders, abdominals, thighs, and feet. Hold for three to five seconds, then slowly lower your knees to the floor.

Challenge Yourself: Perform the exercise with one leg off the floor to decrease stability and increase core-muscle activation.

	Week 13	Week 14	Week 15	Week 16
Reps	10	10	10	10
Sets	1–2	2	2–3	3

3. Abdominal Crisscross

This emphasizes the obliques to strengthen trunk flexion and rotation and increases hamstring length.

1. Lie on your back with your knees bent, feet flat on floor, and hands gently cupping the back of your head.

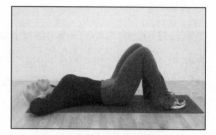

2. Draw in your abdomen, and slowly curl and twist your trunk up as you try to pull your Left knee toward your Right elbow. Reinforce the abdominal contraction, and lower your trunk, elbow, and knee. Repeat on the other side, and alternate in a controlled crisscross pattern.

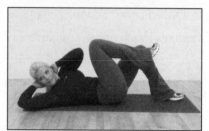

Challenge Yourself: Perform the exercise with your feet on the stability ball, legs straight. Try to keep the ball still.

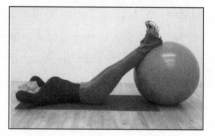

	Week 13	Week 14	Week 15	Week 16
Reps	10	10	10	10
Sets	1–2	2	2–3	3

4. Ticktock

This incorporates abdominals, chest, gluteals, and thighs to control trunk rotation.

1. Lie back, shoulders on the ball, arms outstretched, and palms sandwiched together and pointing upward.

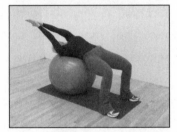

2. Draw in your abdomen, and slowly rotate arms, trunk, and hips to the Right to the two o'clock position.

3. Return to the starting position. Then draw in your abdomen, and slowly rotate arms, trunk, and hips to the Left to the ten o'clock position. Repeat the ticktock motion with a controlled speed.

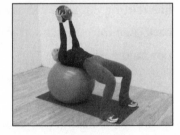

Challenge Yourself: Perform the exercise while holding a medicine ball.

	Week 13	Week 14	Week 15	Week 16
Reps	10	10	10	10
Sets	1–2	2	2–3	3

171

5. Jackknife

This incorporates abdominals, chest, shoulders, arms, and hip flexors to control trunk flexion and resist trunk extension.

1. Lie on your stomach over the stability ball with your hands on the floor. Roll out to a point where your thighs are still on the ball and your feet are off the floor.

2. Draw in your abdomen, and slowly raise your hips toward the ceiling by squeezing your abdominals and pulling your knees forward.

3. Slowly lower your body to a straight-line starting position. Do not arch your back! Reinforce the abdominal contraction, and repeat.

Challenge Yourself: Perform the exercise pulling your knees even closer to your elbows as you lift your buttocks even higher.

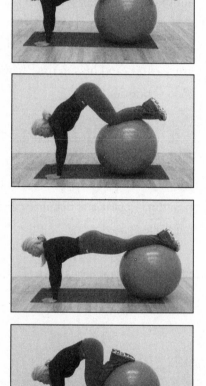

	Week 13	Week 14	Week 15	Week 16
Reps	10	10	10	10
Sets	1–2	2	2–3	3

6. Biceps Curl

This incorporates abdominals, lower back, thighs, and ankles to stabilize the lower body to provide a rigid frame to strengthen the biceps.

1. Sit on the stability ball with your back straight, arms dropped at your sides holding dumbbells, and feet flat on the floor.

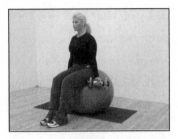

2. Draw in your abdomen, keeping your trunk still, and bend your elbows to curl both dumbbells up to your shoulders. Keep your elbows at your sides, and slowly lower the dumbbells to the starting position. Repeat, keeping your body as still as possible.

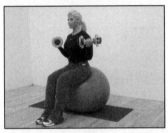

Challenge Yourself: Perform the exercise sitting on the ball while marching (see exercise 4 of Phase 2), keeping your trunk still.

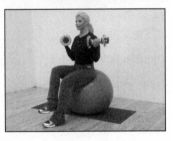

	Week 13	Week 14	Week 15	Week 16
Reps	10	10	10	10
Sets	1–2	2	2–3	3

7. Chest Press

This incorporates abdominals, lower-back muscles, gluteals, and thighs to strengthen the chest, triceps, and shoulders.

1. Lie on your back over the stability ball with your outstretched arms holding dumbbells straight overhead. Your middle and lower back should be supported on top of the ball, and your feet should be resting flat on the floor, shoulder width apart.

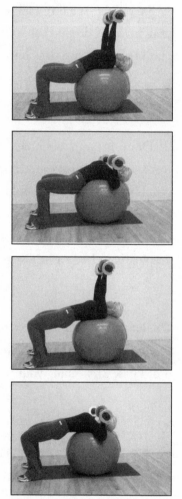

2. Slowly lower the dumbbells, keeping your elbows close to your sides, until the dumbbells flank your head and your elbows are bent fully. Squeeze your chest muscles, and push the dumbbells back to the starting position. Repeat.

Challenge Yourself: Perform the exercise with only your shoulders on the ball, lifting your buttocks in the air to increase your core-muscle activation.

	Week 13	Week 14	Week 15	Week 16
Reps	10	10	10	10
Sets	1–2	2	2–3	3

8. Standing Reverse Flys

This incorporates the lower-back stabilizers, ankles, gluteals, and hamstrings to stabilize the pelvis and trunk to strengthen the upper back, biceps, and postural muscles.

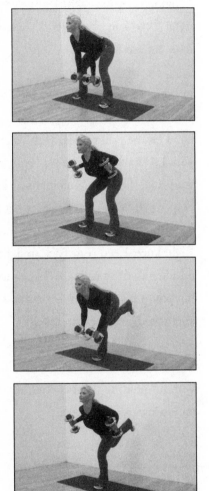

1. Bend forward from the hips a minimum of 45 degrees with a straight back, head straight, legs slightly bent, arms dropped straight down and holding dumbbells.

2. Draw in your abdomen, and squeeze your shoulder blades together. Raise your arms up, focusing on the shoulder-blade squeeze, until your elbows are level with your shoulders. Be sure to keep your back straight, and do not swing your body. Return to the starting position, and repeat.

Challenge Yourself: Perform the exercise standing on one leg.

	Week 13	Week 14	Week 15	Week 16
Reps	10	10	10	10
Sets	1–2	2	2–3	3

9. Single-Leg Squat

This incorporates trunk, ankle, and hip stability to strengthen the thighs and gluteals to improve lower-body balance and strength.

1. Stand on your Right leg, Left foot off the floor, Left knee bent to 90 degrees, Right hand on a wall.

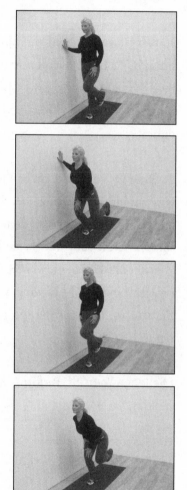

2. Draw in your abdomen, and slowly lower your buttocks in a sitting position, using your hand on the wall to help with balance. Reach your Left hand toward your Right knee. Keep your knee from wobbling from side to side. Stop when your Right knee is bent to about 45 degrees and your Left hand touches your Right knee. Keep your back straight, focusing on hinging from the hip. Return to the starting position, and repeat. After ten repetitions, alternate to the opposite side.

Challenge Yourself: Perform the exercise without holding on to a wall, reaching both hands toward the knee.

	Week 13	Week 14	Week 15	Week 16
Reps	10	10	10	10
Sets	1–2	2	2–3	3

10. Diagonal Chops with Knee Lift

This incorporates the entire body (abdominals, hips, thighs, gluteals, and upper body) to improve speed and coordination of movement in multiple planes. It's also a challenge to endurance to try to maintain intensity for this last exercise.

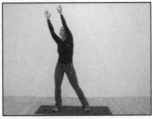

1. Stand with your feet slightly more than shoulder width apart, your trunk turned to the Right and your arms reaching over your head.

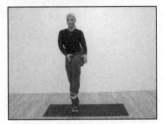

2. Draw in your abdomen, turn your trunk to the Left, and pull your arms down quickly and to the Left as you lift your Left knee up and to the Right. Make sure your trunk remains upright. Return quickly to the starting position with good balance. Repeat with speed. After ten repetitions alternate to the opposite side.

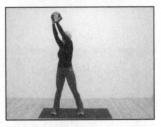

Challenge Yourself: Perform the exercise while holding a medicine ball, or increase your speed without sacrificing technique.

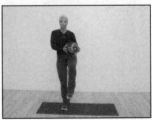

	Week 13	Week 14	Week 15	Week 16
Reps	10	10	10	10
Sets	1–2	2	2–3	3

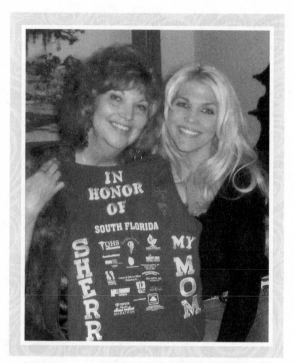

I dedicated my first marathon, in 2005, to my mom.

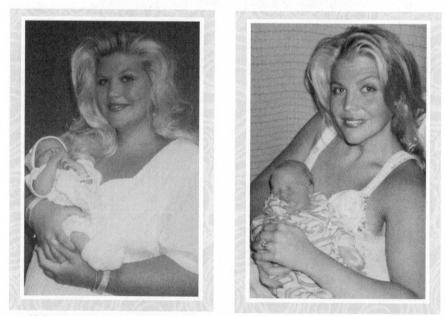

Real life isn't always how we plan it...like getting pregnant. I'm a heavy and out-of-shape new mommy with Kayla in 1996. Then with Luke in 2003, fit and healthy. So much easier!

Chapter 11

Phase 5
Make It Real

Week 17—Eternity

Your Goal:
to make your daily life choices match your desire to be free from diets forever.

What You'll Need to Have
- Exercise equipment to go with your training plans
- A scale and measuring tape

What You'll Need to Know
- By making the decision to change your brain, you have all you need to never let yourself off the hook again!

What You'll Need to Do

- Memorize your Five Decisions.
- Set new goals for yourself.
- Reward yourself regularly.
- Customize your personal eating plan and exercising program.
- Weigh weekly and measure monthly.
- Fill out the self-evaluation in this chapter, and keep it close at hand.

———

You've made it! Sixteen weeks and you are a new person in so many ways. I know it can be easy to second-guess your transformation and live in fear that you'll go back to your old habits, but I'm confident that you really get this. No matter where you are in the weight-loss part of your program, at the end of four months, you should be thinking like a new person. Working out and eating right should no longer be a struggle. If they are, consider redoing Phases 3 and 4. There's no downside to doing this; you can keep on doing those phases forever if they suit your lifestyle well!

Use this week to do a little soul searching. Here are a few signs that you are ready to make this transformation last for the rest of your life:

- You have exercised five days a week almost every week of the past four months.
- You are eating five minimeals of Premium Fuel a day and are keeping your daily calories below 1,500 at least six days a week.
- You can go to a baby shower the day after you have enjoyed an indulgent meal, snack on vegetables instead of petits fours and cake, and feel empowered instead of deprived.
- You are sold on the fact that you will never, ever, as long as you are breathing on this planet, need to go on another diet again.

If that description sounds like you, then welcome to Phase 5!

Now is the time to stop taking directions from me. We're taking off the training wheels and sending you out on your own! That's why Phase 5 is where you make it real. It's about making your fitness plan fit your real life, and it's all up to you. Your workouts, your eating plan, your motivational strategies—you decide what works and what doesn't. I'll leave you with some final advice, but you now have all the tools and knowledge you need to do it on your own.

Don't overthink this stuff. It's normal to be concerned that you've still got a long way to go. Truth be told, I still have those thoughts! In many ways, feeling like that will give you the edge you need to remain on the journey. Becoming too comfortable can make you slack.

One question people keep asking once they get fit is, "What if I have a day when I feel like I'm going to lose control of my eating?" Trust me, you will have those days. I do. When it happens, try to figure out what's really going on. If you're ready to pull on your "Will Kill for Chocolate" T-shirt, maybe monthly hormones are driving the craving. Or maybe this is the day when your precious children have been taken over by aliens bent on destroying the world, starting with your living room. No doubt that's stressful, but eating is not the answer. Neither is food the answer for boredom. In fact, food has never fixed anything other than hunger.

You are bound to have roller-coaster days. Have a plan ready in advance. First, try to get away from food. Plant some flowers, go to a park and walk, listen to music, clean out a closet, have a long workout, call some friends and catch up, read a book to your kids. Just don't try new recipes for the Perfect Chocolate Chip Cookie.

Being in control is more than a feeling; it's about your actions. Sometimes you need to take control by recognizing the signs that you might lose it, and you need to find a way out before it happens. Staying in control the majority of the time will come directly from implementing the Five Decisions that you made a few months ago. When you feel yourself weakening or questioning your commitment to health and fitness, the Five Decisions should be a reminder and checkpoint. They are drilled into my head and stamped on my heart. I must be truthful, forgiving, committed, always interested, and totally surrendered to be the very best I can be in all areas of my life. Without reminding myself of this from time to time, I run the risk of going back to the miserable, hopeless woman I once was. No thanks! I've tasted what life is like on the other side, and the past can't compare!

> Being in control is more
> than a feeling; it's about
> your actions.

Like me, you now own the mind-set for future success in every area of your life. That is the message of *Never Say Diet*. Over the years that I have shared my story with people, I have been asked how I *really* lost the weight. As if I've been keeping it a secret! I always tell people, "I had to stop limiting my life based on what others thought I was capable of and start embracing what God has given me the ability to do." God made me a person who can be the very best I can be every day. He made you to be that kind of person as well. By putting this truth into practice each day, I've had no limitations imposed by outside circumstances.

This program was never intended to be a weight-loss plan alone. Shedding pounds was a priority for me and you, but now we really get it. If you can transform your brain and take control of your body, then you can make just about any dream come true. Press on and set new goals, whether you want to continue losing weight, run your first 5K, or accomplish anything else. You should have already had lots of peak moments along the way, so get ready for many more.

FINALLY, FITNESS FOR A LIFETIME

Phase 5 is where real life begins, even if you are still working on achieving your weight-loss goals. And real life means things don't go as smoothly as you plan. That's why part of your plan has to include staying flexible enough to roll with the punches.

When it comes to doing that, my mother is my hero and my model. As I've mentioned, she has been in a fight of her own for several years. She was diagnosed with leukemia in 1992, then went into remission. Eleven years later she was rediagnosed only weeks after my son Luke was born. She went into remission again. Two years later the cancer was back, and the prognosis was terrible. As I write this, she has shocked all the doctors who have treated her. She is well and full of life, enjoying every minute!

Why has my mother been able to overcome the odds? I ask this all the time. Recently, when she went for a checkup and received an awesome report from her hematologist, it became more obvious to me. My mother has never once complained or asked, "Why is this happening to me?" She has never said, "I'm done fighting. I give up." She just marches like a soldier led by incredible faith that she can face anything with God by her side and the love and support of her family and friends.

I have been guilty of worrying about so many details in my life, obsessing about where I need to be, what I should say, how I look, whether my kids are getting enough vitamins, and whether they'll like a gift I bought for them. I thought about how silly some of this was in comparison to what could occupy my mom's thoughts and discussions, and yet she refuses to allow it. What a lesson for me.

From time to time, we need to clean the lenses through which we view our lives. I pray that *Never Say Diet* has done this for you. While I continued to lose weight, there were still vacations, business trips, sick kids, my own occasional illness, birthday parties, romantic dinners, and unexpected disasters too. Your life will have much of the same. Life, as we all know, does not go according to plan. Being the best you can be doesn't rule out setbacks and crises, but it does set a great standard for dealing with them. When I look at my mom, I get this! She was being the best patient she could be, and the best mother, by setting an example of true faith.

YOUR PROGRESS TO THIS POINT

When my clients reach Phase 5, they often start to wonder what their proper weight should be and how they will know when they get there. To be honest, there isn't a fixed number. Some health and fitness experts try to give one,

Be Passionate About What You Do

Karaoke has completely taken over my parents' lives. This is not a joke. Even their car is wired so they can sing while they travel. And they travel a lot. Several times a year they drive from South Florida to Gatlinburg, Tennessee—their favorite place to visit. When they get there, it's a karaoke-fest every night. They even bring their own CDGs—compact discs with graphics. And when they are home, my parents' schedule is like a rock star's. They stay out some nights until 2 a.m. singing, go home, sleep a little, work, nap, and do it all over again. As if that isn't enough, they have taken up being KJs—karaoke jockeys. For the past several years, every family function has a show to go along with it, no charge.

The greatest part is that they are really good! And I'm not just saying this because they are my parents. When they walk into the local coffee-house, even the young kids start requesting certain songs. I'm amazed, which has always seemed artificial to me. There is usually about a 5-pound range you should try to stay within. Let your body and brain tell you what it is instead of modeling your life after a fashion magazine or the latest Hollywood sensation. If a target weight requires that you starve yourself, it isn't the right number.

Your body is unique to you and can't be manipulated to look exactly like some model or actress. Even if you duplicated every bite of food they eat and every exercise they perform, it wouldn't happen. You shouldn't necessarily look like your high-school self either! Choose a target weight that makes sense for where you are in life today.

In order to keep my fitness plan flexible enough to accommodate the ups and downs of real life, I stick to the 80/20 rule: I follow my eating and workout

but even more I'm grateful that they took this up after I left home. It's the constant practicing that would have driven me insane. For years I thought, *How could they waste so much time doing this one thing?* And then I saw the light. My parents are in love with feeling good about something they are good at. Who isn't? The bonus is that they get praise for doing something they enjoy. People cheer, holler, and clap like crazy—especially when my dad does Johnny Cash. Then they sing a duet and look into each other's eyes like they just met a week ago, and after forty years that's pretty cool too.

I challenge you to live with passion, like my parents, and to make sure you're having fun along the way. Laughter is a key to success and longevity. Play practical jokes, act a little silly, try not to be too serious. You can set a high standard for living while having a blast!

routines 80 percent of the time and go with the flow the other 20 percent. It works well for me, and I encourage you to try it. Be smart, and don't blow your free meals on the first day of the week. Use them for all the stuff in life that's fun: dinner parties, birthday celebrations, holidays, special lunches, brunches, baby showers, and whatever else you choose. You will be able to enjoy these times fully because you maintained healthy eating for the majority of the week, so there is no guilt, and neither is there cheating. (Remember, you decided to forgive yourself and to tell yourself the truth.)

However, you are not me. Your life is your own, so I encourage you to tailor your plan to suit your lifestyle. If it works for you, take off one day entirely, and then eat the other six days as you have practiced. This will obviously depend on whether you have reached your weight goal. If you want to keep losing weight, you'll need to be more rigid and save the indulgences for the future. Whatever you do, always plan ahead. If you do have a setback, simply get back on track the next day or the next meal. Never panic or get discouraged. That's what sends people toward ridiculous desperation diets.

PHASE 5 SELF-EVALUATION

As part of your final preparation to head off into your new life, take time to answer these questions. Then use the wisdom contained in your answers to guide your future decisions.

1. What is the most valuable thing you have learned about yourself in the past sixteen weeks?

2. What is the most valuable thing you have learned about nutrition?

3. What is the most valuable thing you have learned about exercise?

4. What is one three-month goal you have at this time?

5. What is one twelve-month goal you have at this time?

6. What is one dream you have always had that you now think you can make happen?

7. What will it take for you to do this?

8. What area of your life still needs improvement?

9. What ways are you willing to commit to getting better in this area?

10. Finally, I believe we are happiest in life when we are doing for others. The past several months, of necessity, have been about you. Now ask yourself who in your life you can help. Who can you share your change with? Remember, enthusiasm is contagious!

PART THREE

Live

Chapter 12

What You Need to Know About Real Weight Loss

Your Questions Answered with Nothing Held Back

I t sounds so easy…work out, eat right, lose weight, be happy. However, as I discovered, and as I'm sure you know by now, the realities and psychology of getting fit are a lot more complicated than that. There were many things, both during my weight-loss journey and after I'd achieved my goal, that I had to figure out myself. I wish someone had talked to me straight about these things before I had to deal with them on my own. In this chapter we'll talk straight about questions I had as well as questions other people have asked me. I hope it helps you on your journey.

What's the best time of day to do my cardio?

The time that you can make it happen! The main benefits come from consistently doing your cardio, period. You will get results and be burning calories no matter when you do it. However, in a perfect world, the first thing in the morning on an empty stomach is best. The reason is pretty simple. After you have been sleeping for several hours, your body has processed the previous day's food. As you start to exercise, you need fuel to proceed, so your body must turn to your stored fat energy. You burn fat right off the bat! When you do your cardio at other times of the day, you will burn the carbs that you consumed before you will burn fat.

I hate exercise! When did you really start to like it?

I believe the majority of people hate exercise. Most people show up at the gym with a look on their face that says, *I'd rather be having a root canal.* I had been working out for about two months before I started to look forward to it. I think there were two reasons. First, I started getting serious results and started feeling stronger. Second, after two months of exercising and experiencing the "happy drug" endorphins that follow a good workout, I started subconsciously to anticipate them. Overall, I felt less stressed and more in control to deal with other things in life, and I started to really look forward to these feelings.

When working out, should I do the cardio or the strength training first?

This is a question I had for years. I've read a lot of conflicting information about it. If your life allows, doing the cardio first thing on an empty stomach is optimal, as I said earlier. If strength training at the same time is your plan, then do it after the cardio. However, if you're exercising later in the day, after you've had a few meals, do the reverse: strength training, then cardio. If you head to the gym in the afternoon and start with strength training, you burn the day's calories quickly, because it takes more energy to push yourself to finish the sets than it does to move at a steady pace on a treadmill. By the time you proceed to cardio, you'll be burning at a higher rate and will get into your stored fat faster. Hey, if you've got a flexible schedule, doing cardio first thing in the morning and strength training later in the day would be ideal. I know, you're thinking, *Yeah right, dream on!*

Should I get a personal trainer, and did you have one?

Having a "personal" anything is a luxury. No one needs a personal trainer, though I won't deny trainers can be great. If you can afford it and you think it will help you, go for it. I have never had a personal trainer. But I have been blessed along the way by meeting lots of experts who have shared so much advice with me, some of which is found in this book. One useful thing about a trainer is that she can help you cut through the conflicting information you're bound to get. If you decide to hire a trainer along with committing to the Brain-Change program, make sure the trainer understands your plan and supports it. Pay attention to the method of training that she uses as well. Just pushing fixed weight on a machine for all your workouts is not useful for real-life movements, as I discussed in Phase 2.

I actually love my daily exercise. My problem is that I am so hungry afterward. Did this happen to you, and how did you balance this when you were trying to lose weight?

I learned about this as I became more fit. When I started, my body had plenty of stored fat, so I didn't experience true hunger as much in the beginning. But by the time I was training for a marathon, I would get ravenous. The key is to schedule your meals appropriately. By having a solid meal with protein and complex carbs no more than thirty minutes after you finish exercising, you will help avoid uncontrollable hunger. When you work out and rev up your engine, it needs fuel right away. If you wait too long, you create a problem: your blood sugar drops, you get the shakes, and you get hungry and irritable. And then you work hard to bring your blood sugar back up by eating, and you risk eating too many calories. Eating protein just after a workout also repairs and builds muscle more effectively than eating it hours later.

I can't wait to get this weight off. Why don't I eat 1,000 calories a day instead of 1,500?

Believe me, I felt exactly that way early on. But I need to say one more time, if rapid weight loss is your main goal, this program is not right for you. If you eat only 1,000 calories a day, you set yourself up for rebounds and long-term failure. Permanent weight loss should not be too rapid. Think about it; did you go on a rapid weight-gaining program? Probably not. It was a process of bad habits that produced weight gain over time. Think about this as reversing the process. If you eat too few calories, it won't be long before you will be undernourished and underenergized, because your metabolism will have slowed. You may not have many friends either, because you'll be so grumpy. Realistically, this is a setup for serious disappointment. You don't want another diet; you want a new lifestyle that just happens to make you healthy, trim, and fit. Don't worry; it will happen, and you'll enjoy the process a lot more.

I have been doing great, and then yesterday I fell apart at lunch. I felt guilty and then ate out of control for the rest of the day. Is this a disaster? How can I stop it from happening again?

This kind of behavior is normal for a lot of people. The mistake would be to continue to have a diet mentality. Since you are creating a new lifestyle and there is no finish line, one bad lunch shouldn't ruin your day. Think about it this way: if you back out of your driveway and hit the mailbox, you stop, set the parking brake, assess the damage, and go. You continue with your day. You don't keep backing into the mailbox over and over just because you hit it once. Blowing the rest of your day by going on an eating frenzy is like that. Everybody makes mistakes. Move on.

I've had so many food-heavy work functions and parties lately, and I feel like I'm cheated out of celebrating. I end up not wanting to attend these events. Did you deal with this, do you have any suggestions, and are you going to tell me to just suck it up?

Yes, yes, and pretty much. I did deal with this and continue to. It's stressful. My suggestion is to eat healthy food before the event and to have a nonnegotiable rule that you won't touch food at the event. If you show up hungry, you'll start picking, and soon you'll have picked up a crazy amount of calories. Also, figure out what is being served that you can have, and fill up on that before you weaken. If you suspect that you won't find anything acceptable to eat at the event, have a plan. Decide in advance when you will leave and what you will eat. If it's a chicken breast and sweet potato, you'll really look forward to it. As far as sucking it up goes, sometimes you have to. Don't eat a little of your favorite things when you are in a weight-loss phase. It's easy to break down quickly. On the other hand, don't skip the events just because you fear the food. That's just another way of letting food rule your life.

I know people who have lost weight by not eating carbs. Do I really need some, and if so, how many grams is right to do the job and still make the scale go down?

No-carb diets work at first because almost all the big calorie bombs involve carbs. How much meat, oil, and veggies can you really pack away? But we now know why no-carb diets don't work down the line. Once you bring the carbs back—and there's no way to eat normally without them—your body doesn't know how to burn them efficiently. Your energy and metabolism are shot. You're then on the fast track to weight gain. How many carbs you need a day to keep your fires burning bright depends on how much weight you need to lose and your current body fat. For me, starting out at more than 50 percent body fat, I had enough to survive the great Y2K famine of 2000, which didn't show up, so I had to simulate one. I stuck to under 100 grams (400 calories) of carbs per day for my first 100 pounds of weight loss. Then, as I lost body fat, I needed more carbs to provide energy and still lose weight. So I increased to 150 grams (600 calories) of carbs per day, remaining at 1,500 total calories a day.

What do you think is the worst possible thing we can eat?

Trans fats. They are so damaging that New York City recently banned all trans fats from its restaurants. Trans fats have the worst impact of any nutrient on your cholesterol, meaning they contribute to heart attacks, strokes, diabetes, and all the other cardiovascular diseases. Trans fats are made by taking normal, liquid vegetable oil and bubbling hydrogen gas through it until it turns solid at room temperature. (Crisco and margarine are perfect examples.) The oil doesn't spoil as quickly, so it extends the shelf life of crackers, cookies, and baked goods. Fast-food restaurants and companies that sell prepackaged items in grocery stores love trans fats but now are reworking recipes to find alternatives. Still, we are a long way from being rid of them. The words for you to look for on ingredients lists are *hydrogenated* or *partially hydrogenated.*

What is "good fat"? I thought all fat was bad.

So did nutritionists and researchers back in the eighties and nineties. Many people still act on that misinformation! Fats have more than twice as many calories per gram as do protein and carbohydrates, so if you ate the same amount of fat as of protein or carbs, you'd be eating way too many calories. But when was the last time you consumed a slab of butter the size of a chicken breast or a glass of olive oil the size of a soft drink? Fat is so rich that we tend to eat it in small amounts, and it diminishes appetite, so the current wisdom is that carbs, not fat, are the big culprit in most weight gain. Fat was also thought to raise bad cholesterol and clog the arteries, but now we know that only saturated fat—the kind that comes from animals and is solid at room temperature—and trans fats do that. Unsaturated fat—found in fish, olive oil, vegetable oils, and nuts—improves your cholesterol and, in moderation, is one of the healthiest nutrients you can eat.

Just before I have my period, I have a strong need for chocolate. So I'm wondering: once I have my sugar issues under control, is this okay once in a while?

Believe it or not, chocolate can be good for you. Dark chocolate—look for a minimum of 60 percent cocoa content on the label—is packed with antioxidants that can cut your risk of cardiovascular disease. Just consume no more than two ounces at a time as one of your two snacks, which should cut the craving without adding too many calories.

Some of my girlfriends started out so supportive but now have begun to treat me differently. Do you know what I mean?

I could write an entire book on the dynamics of friendship and the different reasons we choose certain people to be in our lives. When it comes to women and weight loss, my experience—and others have confirmed this—is that people who are smaller than you are very excited for you at first. "Keep it up!" they say. Then as you get closer to their size, they hold back on the compliments: "Now, I hope you aren't starving yourself." Once you are even with them, it's "You're not trying to lose any more weight, are you?" And once you pass them, the daggers really come out.

Learn from my mistake: don't offer these people the clothes that are now too big for you. In general, remember that you can't control how people react to you; you can only control your reaction. An "it's all good" mentality will save your hurt feelings. Remind yourself that you've got something going on inside that they may wish they had.

Why do the last 10 pounds seem the hardest to lose?

You may have chosen an unrealistic number for your target weight. If you are fit and are eating right but the scale has stopped dropping, you may be at your natural healthy weight. Being your best isn't defined by a number on a scale. Remember that there is no one precise number to obsess about. We all naturally fluctuate within a range of about 5 pounds. By decreasing your daily food intake below 1,500 calories, you can probably push beyond your natural healthy weight to an arbitrary number you've picked. But it will eventually make you depressed. On the other hand, maybe you have crept back to a lifestyle where you are indulging a little more than you should. If that's the case, you might want to go back to Phase 4, be strict, and see if that makes the difference.

I've reached my target weight, but now I'm pregnant. Should I stop my workouts and my eating plan, and how much weight is okay to gain during my pregnancy?

That pretty much happened to me. Remember, the mission doesn't change. Being the best pregnant woman you can be is your plan for the next nine months. After clearing this with your ob-gyn, you should continue to work out and maintain a healthy eating plan. Let your hunger be your guide; just don't stop at every Dairy Queen you pass. Most doctors recommend that you gain between 25 and 35 pounds if you are at a normal starting weight. By the way, congratulations!

I injured myself, and I can't work out for a while. I'm scared I'm going to gain all my weight back.

Most people who are active will experience an injury at some point. Explain your situation to your doctor, and see if he or she can recommend any alternative exercises. Plenty of cardiovascular exercises, such as swimming, are low impact and often can be done while you recover from injuries. As far as the potential for gaining weight, you will need to be careful. Because you are not burning as many calories, you need to make adjustments accordingly. On the upside, you will also not be as hungry.

Now that I've reached my weight goal, I miss the excitement of watching the scale go down. What should I do?

I know this feeling well. It is addictive! Let your excitement now come from other things that are measurable. For me, it was seeing how much money I could raise for leukemia research as well as completing marathons and improving my running times.

I, too, have always dreamed of running a marathon. How should I get started?

Know this first: running a marathon is not a weight-loss program! In fact, it's important that you clear up food issues beforehand, because as you run more and more, you want to eat everything in sight. You can even justify it in your mind because of the long workouts. I have seen people actually put on weight this way. Once you are maintaining your weight, however, running a marathon can be a major life accomplishment. If you are serious, you will want to find a training program that works for your schedule and then enter a race. Better yet, consider training with a group for a special cause. You will have access to experienced coaching, team spirit to keep you going, and the fulfillment of doing something for others. Team In Training is an awesome organization that

I am proud to be a coach with. They are responsible for raising millions of dollars each year to help find a cure for leukemia, lymphoma, and other cancers.

What are the best shoes for my workouts?

If only I had found the answer before training for my first marathon cost me eight toenails! The best sneakers are the ones that best fit your feet and have a design that aids in correcting the way you naturally land when you walk or run. I love Asics; to me they are the best shoes on the planet, especially for running. However, you may find that another brand better fits your feet. Try to find someone in the store who can do a gait analysis to help you determine what you need in a shoe.

My teenage daughter is overweight. How can I approach her?

This is a difficult one. First, you need to know your daughter. If she is open about her weight, take her out for a walk, and tell her that you want to help. Use this book, and get her interested in making lifelong decisions to improve her health. I'm not above offering incentives as motivation, like new clothes.

If your daughter seems embarrassed to discuss her weight, like I was, you face a bigger challenge. The thing to do is to bring up the topic without making her feel like you are judging her. An approach based on "I just want you to be healthy" will turn her off fast. You may find that saying something like, "I'm so glad my diet days are over!" will lead to a meaningful discussion about my story and this book. Sharing your personal battle with weight and body image will help her relate to you. No matter what you say or do, this is going to be hard and may not spark change immediately. Lord knows my mother tried in many ways, yet I didn't do anything until I was ready, at age twenty-nine. The following chapter will give you additional ideas. Just don't give up.

I am losing weight, and my husband is gaining it! Why can't I make him do this with me?

Probably for the same reason that my husband hates taking my Spinning classes—because it's your idea. All I can really say is keep on keeping on. While I understand that you want him to lose weight and become fit, the desire needs to come from within him. However, make sure that the food you put on the table is solid and premium most of the time. If he wants to eat poorly, let him find it for himself. And please don't have him call me!

As I am losing weight, the skin on my face is changing. What can I do about it?

People who tend to be heavy or store weight in their face often have pretty skin. It is the fat cells that make it full and supple. As you lose weight, you lose volume in your face, and then you have too much skin covering too little area. It can be aggravating when your skin starts to look worse as your body looks better. I've found a few things that help: stay hydrated by drinking lots of water, minimize time in the sun (I love self-tanners), and use a moisturizer nearly every hour on the hour!

My stomach is the worst part of my body. Can I do sit-ups every day?

Yes. But remember that nearly every exercise in this book is already geared toward strengthening your core, which includes your abs. Also, if you have layers of fat on your stomach, you can do two hundred sit-ups a day, and you won't look tight and flat. As you lose weight and continue strength training, you will eventually see results there.

If I have a cold, should I still exercise?

The rule that I think makes the most sense is this: if your symptoms are from the neck up only, then yes. But if they are below your neck, such as congestion in your lungs, take a little break and get well. A fever is definitely a reason to lie low. Allowing your body to fight a possible infection is important. And, as always, stay well hydrated.

Is there a serious difference between exercising in a regular bra and a sports bra?

Absolutely. When you wear a regular bra, even one with good support, it is usually not enough to keep your breasts from moving too much when you exercise. A sports bra is designed with more coverage; therefore it provides more support. Many women who always thought of exercise as uncomfortable discover that a sports bra makes a huge difference. Make sure you get one that fits well and is tight enough to do a good job but still allows you to breathe.

I don't sweat when I exercise. Is this normal?

It might be for you. Definitely not for me. I once thought I had a yet-to-be-diagnosed sweat disease! Don't forget that sweating is your body's way to cool down when its internal temperature gets too high. Sweating is very healthy, and some people are more active sweaters than others. Don't worry too much about it. Just be sure to drink enough water to replace what you're losing, especially if you live in a dry climate. Most people think that high humidity makes us sweat more, but the humidity actually just makes it harder for the sweat to evaporate from our skin, so it tends to accumulate. If you live in Arizona, you may be sweating plenty while you exercise and not even realize it.

I have heard about liposuction but don't really know how it works. Could you explain it to me, and do you think it's helpful?

Liposuction is a surgical procedure that removes fat out of specific areas of the body. The myth is that this can make you skinny. Because fat is stored throughout our bodies, it is impossible to lipo it all. Even if it were possible, it would be extremely unhealthy. You need your fat cells for all sorts of body processes; you just don't need all the fat stored in those cells. But lipo removes your natural cells along with the fat. More important, lipo doesn't improve your health. The one major study that has been done found that people who removed 20 pounds of fat through lipo still had all the cardiovascular problems they had before. However, people who made the right dietary and exercise changes improved their cholesterol, blood pressure, and blood sugar *almost immediately,* before any real weight had come off.[9] It's clear that the health benefits come not from changing a number on a scale but from retraining your body to start burning fat again. Lipo can be useful in certain cases, if performed after weight loss to address a resistant area—for instance, saddlebags that won't go away.

And what about body sculpting?

Body sculpting, according to Leonard Hochstein, MD, a prominent Miami Beach plastic surgeon, is a more sophisticated procedure that achieves better results than lipo.[10] If you simply lipo out the fat underlying the skin, the skin loses its padding and tends to look concave and sickly. This is especially true for people who have lost a lot of weight, because the skin was stretched so far that it has already lost a lot of its elasticity. Body sculpting combines lipo with skin excision to tighten the skin against the body and restore its tone. Again, it only makes sense after you've lost weight on your own.

I don't want my breasts to get smaller as I lose weight. Are there any exercises I can do to concentrate the weight loss on my thighs?

If there were any exercises that worked like this, plastic surgeons would be driving Toyotas. Breasts are made up of fat tissue. Different body types store fat differently. But no matter who you are, as you start to shed pounds, fat comes off all over, and that means your breasts will shrink. Strength training will improve the look of your body and is meant to both tighten and tone it. And building more chest muscle can increase your bust measurement slightly. But that's about all you can do naturally.

How did you decide it was time to consider plastic surgery yourself?

I honestly did not consider any surgery until I had my last child, more than three years into my transformation. Once I had maintained my weight loss and continued to get even more fit, I realized I had excess skin that had lost its elasticity and wasn't going back, and there was nothing I could do myself to change that. I decided to have a breast lift and augmentation, and this was a difficult decision. I understand that we need to accept our bodies as God created them, but God did not intend for me to balloon up to 350 pounds. There were ramifications from this that I knew could be fixed. I fixed everything I could through clean eating and exercise, then got help from experts for what I couldn't do on my own.

Did you discuss having plastic surgery with your husband and family? How have they reacted?

Yes, I discussed it with my husband first and then my mom and daughters. I wanted them to understand the frustration of losing a lot of weight, becoming superfit, and then being disappointed with my body as a result. They were incredibly supportive and understood this was not simply vanity. But as I moved forward with this decision, I wanted to consider the message I was sending my children. I wanted my girls to know their mom was fixing a problem that she had created herself, that this was not simply a matter of wanting bigger breasts.

What is the message you most want to send about plastic surgery?

That it is important to be realistic. Plastic surgery does not make you lean, give you a new body shape, or cause you to drop two sizes. It does not give you lifelong good health. On the other hand, it has helped give many people the life they wanted. Plastic surgery should be viewed as a personal choice and an option to enhance the work you have already done.

Dr. Joseph Capella is a plastic surgeon who specializes in working with people who have had significant weight loss. He is considered one of the top surgeons in the country in this field, so I went to him for authoritative answers.

Dr. Capella, how can a person know when she has lost enough weight to start considering plastic surgery?

Because plastic surgery is not designed to aid in weight loss, it is important that you get to your goal weight or set point first. Once you have achieved this, you will want to have stayed within a few pounds of that number for at least six months. This will ensure the best possible results.

Dr. Capella, what questions should a woman ask if she is trying to choose a plastic surgeon?

Perhaps the most important question to ask is whether the surgeon is board certified in plastic surgery specifically. Body contouring after weight loss is a relatively new area within the field of plastic surgery, and therefore it is important to know how much experience the surgeon has with this patient population.

Some questions you might ask include:

- How many of these procedures do you perform each month?
- Are postoperative photographs available of other patients who have undergone these procedures?
- Would it be possible to speak with patients who have recently undergone these procedures?

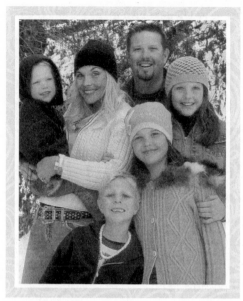

My family (from left): Luke, Jake, Kayla, Keith, Ashley

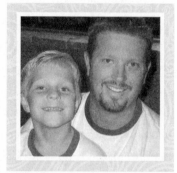

My husband, Keith, with our older son, Jake

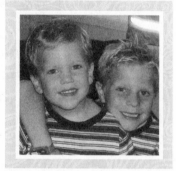

My boys, Luke and Jake

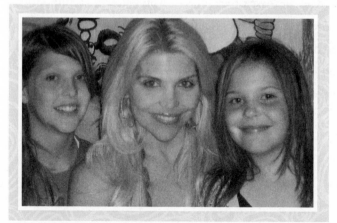

Me with my girls, Ashley and Kayla

Chapter 13

Five Ways to Get Your Family Fit

It's Never Too Soon to Start

This book wouldn't be complete if it talked only about *your* health and fitness. Whatever our situation in life, however young or old we are, all of us want to see those we love thriving. And so our families become our focus.

This subject is very close to my heart. The most obvious reason is that I was an overweight child. Even before I had children, I worried that one day I would watch mine go through the same pain I had experienced and that I wouldn't know how to help them. As each of my children was born, I wondered which would follow in my footsteps. I prayed that they would all escape their genetic doom.

Over the past several years, while making my own transformation, I realized this fear was unnecessary. My children were not doomed to any particular fate. Just as I had control over whether I chose to stay fat and miserable, I also had control of what life lessons about health and fitness I gave my family. I couldn't make every decision for them, but I could help them make good choices. And the best way to instill that behavior would be to model it. I don't believe we earn the right to drill values into our children if we don't live by them ourselves.

As I overheard a group of mothers discussing the importance of which preschool they could get their three-year-olds into, I had a revelation. Even before our children are born, we start planning how best to take care of them. As they start to grow, we plan for their education, help choose their friends, make them do their homework, and try our best to build them into responsible adults. The ironic part is that as we work hard to make sure our kids have the best, we sometimes stop giving them our best.

You probably know the numbers. Childhood obesity rates are soaring. By 2010 half of North America's kids will be overweight. More than a third of those will be truly obese.[11] And teasing is the least of the problems these kids face. Being overweight as a child is a fast track to diabetes, cardiovascular disease, depression, and many other health problems. The upshot of all this is that the current generation of kids is predicted to be the first in history with a *lower* life expectancy than their parents. Unbelievable!

It's not like kids have suddenly become lazy and ungrateful or have developed a new addiction to sweets and video games. The real epidemic is parents who can't say no and stick to it! Parents who overindulge and are underdisciplined pass those traits and habits on to their children. There's no point in talking about getting families fit until we've addressed this first.

We can't blame the fast-food industry, the computers and games, or the lack of physical education in our schools. Our problems stem from us. And this is coming from someone who understands how difficult it is. I've been frazzled when the kids get home from school and need help with homework, and we have to squeeze in visits to the orthodontist, piano lessons, and dinner. Your four-year-old screams for his third Fruit Roll-Up, and when you refuse to give it to him, a scene from *The Exorcist* unfolds. Then the phone rings, and it's your mother-in-law wanting to know why those kids scream all the time, and boy would it be easy just to hand over that Fruit Roll-Up. But by saying no consistently, we teach our kids to save the drama because the drama doesn't work. Then when you do say yes, it has value.

> *Being overweight as a child is a fast track to diabetes, cardiovascular disease, depression, and many other health problems.*

We have no one to blame but ourselves if we have unhealthy kids. Is anyone really surprised that eating a Big Mac every day is bad for you? Or that sitting around all day makes you fat? Doing it to ourselves is inexcusable, but it's even worse to do it to our kids. So what can we do to help our families be fit? Following are some things I do in my home. I know it can be a struggle to stay on top of this. But you and I have decided to be the best we can, and that especially applies to the job of mom, which also happens to give the greatest return.

1. FIGURE OUT THE FLAWS

When you decide to have a healthy home, figure out which areas need improvement. Usually it's a combination of a few things, including not enough exercise or too much junk food. If your kids lie around every afternoon in front of the television with a bag of Doritos, you know it isn't good. Start using the Brain-Change process to become the best parent you can be. Go back to the Five Decisions—to be truthful, forgiving, committed, and interested, and to surrender—and now apply them to this new role. Decide that you will do whatever it takes to teach your family the value of healthy living.

2. Don't Just Preach It; Teach It

Just as you have spent time learning what to eat and how to exercise, now you must take the time to teach it in your home. When your kids ask why they have to stop playing that video game or eating those cookies, have a truthful and meaningful answer ready. Saying "Because I said so!" will encourage them to sneak behind your back because they think you're just being mean. I have found that if I take the time to give my kids information, they don't fight me in their response.

And don't use threats, even ones like "If you eat that, you'll get fat!" Too negative. You don't want to be constantly taking things away and using scare tactics. You want to show that better choices ultimately give us what we want most. Explain how going for a bike ride will help us get nice muscles, how eating this carrot will give us pretty skin and good vision. They'll get the message because you have taught them the long-term value first.

3. Keep Their Choices Clean Too!

Most of us know this, but I still need to mention it. There's nothing wrong with an occasional treat, but a treat isn't a treat if it's an everyday thing. Even if your son is skinny as a rail, junk food still junks up the inside of his body. I know the favorite fruit of my husband and each of my kids. I try to always have it in the house, washed and cut up if need be. Because kids don't do the grocery shopping, you have control over what food choices are available in your home. If the options are chips or celery sticks, any kid is going to pick the chips. But if the only choices are fruits and vegetables, kids will be content with those.

Also, suggest snack ideas that kids can make on their own. Apples with peanut butter, carrots with low-fat dressing, popcorn sprinkled with parmesan, and many more are well within the capabilities of most kids. As far as school lunches go, it's a good idea to pack it most of the time. I love my kids' schools, but I have been in the cafeterias and looked at the menus. For the most part it is overprocessed, mass-quantity food. This is not the quality we want them to get on a regular basis.

4. MAKE MOVEMENT MEANINGFUL

You don't like to feel tortured by exercise, and neither do your kids. And there's no reason for them to be. We are meant to move. It feels good—much better than just sitting around. The problem is that some kids have lost the habit of physical play or were never given the opportunity to develop it. Computers are great, and Game Boys have kept peace and harmony in my car on many occasions, but limits are necessary. Finding balance is the important thing. I've tried hard to introduce family times that make physical activity fun and natural. My kids like to have swimming relays, hula-hoop contests, and their own cheerleading competitions in the living room. By making exercise such as walks, bike riding, hiking, skating, or shooting hoops a family fun time, you're changing up the movie-and-ice-cream afternoons and adding a health benefit.

If you are having trouble finding things that your kids like to do, take them to a sporting goods store and have them look around. You may be surprised what you find. In South Florida outdoor activities are really big, but I never expected ice skating to be one of them. Then, two years ago, my daughter took an interest in it. Now she takes lessons and competes. I know she loves it, and it's a diversion from boredom. Coming from the past I had, I find personal joy in hearing her ask me to take her to practice, even when she is not scheduled to be there.

5. SAYING NO SAYS, "I LOVE YOU"; SAYING YES SAYS IT TOO

God expects us to let our *yes* mean yes and our *no* mean no. When you say, "No, you can't eat that," make sure your kids know that you care, that you limit their options because you love them. In the past I made the mistake of treating discipline as a power trip. I thought it was a chance to show I was the boss, and I usually ended up regretting it. But laying down the law is also part of showing love. God does it with us, and we have a responsibility to do it in our homes. It's not always going to be received in the proper spirit. But by doing what it takes to prevent your children from having serious, preventable health and weight and food issues, you are giving them love for a lifetime.

At the same time, don't forget that saying yes is superimportant as well. Having rewards makes us all want to do better. It doesn't always need to be a Slurpee, but once in a while it's necessary to just be a kid.

ONE MOM'S STORY

I received this e-mail from a client, and I was so inspired by it that I want to share it with you.

> I have been overweight most of my life. For years, I felt out of control and lost sight of who I really was. I have tried so many different diets in my life, only to fail and gain even more weight. I was miserable inside. In January 2007, at age 34, I weighed 328 pounds, which made me sad and angry that I had let myself get to that point. That same month, I had an incident that shook me. I was turned down for per-

sonal health insurance and a life insurance policy due to my excessive weight. I was mortified that I had become so obese that insurance companies wouldn't cover me. I felt broken and hopeless.

That is when I had a divine meeting with Chantel. Listening to her speak, and how her brain worked, changed my life. I realized that it was a matter of a decision on my part. I decided never to be the same again. For the first time in my life, I felt hope and could see the light at the end of the tunnel.

Then I experienced another wake-up call. I had noticed for several years that my seven-year-old daughter's eating habits had become like mine. She loved sweets and always got second helpings. I could see what was happening physically, but I didn't let myself think about it because I was trying to get myself together. During a routine visit to [my daughter's] pediatrician, the doctor looked at me and said, "We have a problem." She informed me that my daughter's weight was that of a teenager. At that moment, I felt like all the air in my lungs had been sucked out. There I was on my journey, losing weight and not paying attention to my precious little girl's health. I blamed myself for this, but I also knew that I now held the key that could help her.

Now my family is sharing in my healthy lifestyle. I know that the same-sex parent is the biggest influencer on a child, so now I am influencing my daughter in a whole new way! I have lost 65 pounds—something I thought I could never do. My daughter is also eating healthy and trimming down. I'm on this journey, no turning back, no option to fail. This is my time to conquer this once and for all, and to teach my kids how to live a lifestyle so they won't have to walk the path that I did. Thank you, Chantel![12]

The Power of Reason

Kids can be surprisingly open to reason. My four-year-old son, Luke, has a ritual at bedtime. We read a story first, then sing a night-night song that I made up when he was a baby, then pray, and then he gets a sippy cup. The drink was mostly water with a little apple juice, but I was worried about sending him to sleep with juice after he'd brushed his teeth, so I tried to break the habit. He threw a tantrum every night. This went on for about two months, and I'd occasionally give in.

Finally I'd had enough. I read him a book where a boy named David tries to become a pirate. The pirates in the illustrations have scary and rotten teeth. I explained to Luke that rotten teeth come from too much sugar and no brushing. I explained that having juice before going to sleep could rot his teeth, and I showed him in a mirror how nice his teeth were. That was it! Each night now he takes his cup and asks, "Mommy, this is water, right? I don't want pirate teeth." If you can be creative when communicating a point with your children, they will usually get it!

Chapter 14

Live with Purpose!

You Are Strong Enough to Finish Anything

Let me tell you about the day of my twenty-mile training run in preparation for my first marathon. When my friend Rob and I set out that morning at four o'clock, I had no idea that we were in for an unforgettable ordeal. We had been training for the Disney Marathon with Team In Training, a branch of the Leukemia and Lymphoma Society.

At the start of our morning run, we were feeling great. By mile ten the sun wasn't quite up, it was cool, we were feeling strong, and it was time to turn around. Our coach, Roy Feifer, came up behind us. Rob and I were both drenched in sweat, but Roy didn't have a drop on him. He was barely breathing hard. "Hey, guys," he said, "I have an idea. Let's go up a little farther, because my friend is going to be proposing to his girlfriend on the beach at sunrise, and we can congratulate them."

I'm a romantic, and this sounded like a must to me. The timing was just right. We went for it. I didn't really consider the extra miles we were adding.

We got to Atlantic Avenue, and all three of us walked out on the sand. We saw a couple huddled under a blanket in the distance and ran toward them. As we got within a few feet, Roy said, "No, that's not them!" Oops. By then, Rob was over the whole thing and wouldn't stop talking about the sand in his shoes. We just kept wandering down the shoreline. Finally Roy spotted his friends. We weren't sure if the big question had been popped yet, and we didn't want to spoil the moment. So we hid behind some trees and watched the perfect sunrise. Minutes later we saw them kiss, and we ran across the sand, yelling, "Congratulations!" Roy hugged his friends, Rob and I introduced ourselves, and then we took off for home. Roy went ahead to check on other teammates while Rob and I kept running at our same pace.

Of course by that time we had added extra miles to our run, and the Florida sun was now high in the sky. We were not prepared for this. A few miles after heading back we both started to fall apart. There was a wall, and we slammed into it! We slowed way down and eventually had to walk the last seven miles in a state of confused dehydration. When we made it back, I was delirious. I was nauseous, my toes were bleeding, and my lower back felt broken. It was the worst run I could have imagined. And this was only a few weeks before the real event—26.2 miles.

I struggled mentally and physically all the next week. I feared I couldn't run the marathon. All the miles and hours I had spent training seemed to have no value. My focus was only on that last brutal training run. I even begged Rob to do another twenty miler with me the following week, hoping we would finish stronger and feel more prepared. But Rob, who's a podiatrist, was smart enough to refuse. I believe his exact words were "You're out of your mind." This was no new revelation, but he said the date of the race was way too close to risk an injury during another long training run. If I ran another twenty miler, I'd be on my own.

*From here on, you can live
your life like you are training
for a marathon.*

So I called Roy, our coach, to plead my case. And he knew exactly what I needed to hear. "It's normal to be nervous, but remember why you are doing this." I knew my motivation was to be a part of the cure for leukemia. He also said, "Remember that a few weeks earlier, you finished that eighteen-mile run singing." He was right. And finally, "Chan, you've put in the time. You've done everything right to be ready for the race. So forget about the bad run, move on, and, trust me, you will finish."

He was right. A couple of weeks later I crossed the finish line feeling like the old me had disappeared that day forever. I knew I would never be the same. And it felt better than I could ever describe. I had put in the time and had laid all the groundwork necessary to become the new me, and there was no way I was going to let one bad run throw me off my purpose.

From here on, you can live your life like you are training for a marathon. Get ready to enjoy peak moments on a regular basis. Tremendous finish-line experiences are worth the discipline and self-control it takes to get there.

You need to trust that you have prepared well. You have invested the last four months getting ready. And just as I had a disastrous twenty-mile training run, you will have setbacks and discouraging days. But remember why you are doing this. And don't forget the peak moments you've had along the way; they will help you stay the course. You are strong enough now to go out and finish anything. And when you hear that some magical moment is happening just up ahead, a little farther than you planned on going, I hope you'll push yourself to experience it. You'll be glad you did. I know I was. I wouldn't trade that sunrise for anything.

I Want to Hear from You!

In this book I've done my best to anticipate your biggest questions and concerns and to give you all the tools you need to achieve lasting weight loss. I hope it has changed your life! If it has, I want to hear about it. And if you have more questions, I want to hear them too. That's why I've set up a Web site to provide ongoing support and to help me stay in touch with everyone who's on the same journey as I am.

Please visit the site to find free downloads, advice, motivational techniques, information on workout clothing and equipment, and other new information. You can also go to the Web site to join an online accountability program, to learn what's new with me, and to share your story with others. I hope to hear from you soon.

www.chantelhobbs.com

Notes

1. Christopher D. Gardner and others, "Comparison of the Atkins, Zone, Ornish, and LEARN Diets for Change in Weight and Related Risk Factors Among Overweight Premenopausal Women: The A to Z Weight Loss Study: A Randomized Trial," *Journal of the American Medical Association,* 297, no. 9 (March 7, 2007): 969–77.

2. "Welcome to L.A. Weight Loss," reported by Samantha M. Wender, broadcast on *20/20,* ABC, February 16, 2007. Transcript available at http://abcnews.go.com/2020/Story?id=2877644&page=1.

3. Eugenia E. Calle and others, "Overweight, Obesity, and Mortality from Cancer in a Prospectively Studied Cohort of U.S. Adults," *New England Journal of Medicine,* 348, no. 17 (April 24, 2004): 1625–38.

4. "Weight Loss and a Healthy Breakfast," Harvard Health Publications, Harvard Medical School, www.health.harvard.edu/press_releases/weight_loss_healthy_breakfast.htm.

5. Holly R. Wyatt and others, "Long-Term Weight Loss and Breakfast in Subjects in the National Weight Control Registry," *Obesity Research* 10 (2002): 78–82.

6. Selene Yeager, "Rev Your Metabolism: Drink Water," *Prevention,* www.prevention.com/article/1,5778,s1-2-67-682-4141-1,00.html.

7. Kirsten A. Burgomaster and others, "Six Sessions of Sprint Interval Training Increases Muscle Oxidative Potential and Cycle Endurance Capacity in Humans," *Journal of Applied Physiology* 98 (2005): 1985–90.

8. Peter Jaret, "A Healthy Mix of Rest and Motion," *New York Times,* May 3, 2007, E1, E8.

9. Gina Kolata, *Rethinking Thin: The New Science of Weight Loss—and the Myths and Realities of Dieting* (New York: Farrar, Straus, and Giroux, 2007), 210–12.

10. From personal e-mail with the author, June 26, 2007.

11. "Childhood Obesity Expected to Soar Worldwide," MSNBC, March 7, 2006, www.msnbc.msn.com/id/11694799.

12. This e-mail message is used with permission of the writer.

The *Never Say Diet* Exercises

The cardio and strength-training program in *Never Say Diet* was designed by Chantel Hobbs in conjunction with Joe Tedesco, DPT, ATC, CSCS, a certified athletic trainer and physical therapist. Joe and his wife, Lesley Tedesco, are doctors of physical therapy at Elite Physical Therapy in Charlotte, North Carolina.

Joe specializes in the treatment of orthopedic and sports physical therapy of the spine and extremities. He also trains clients who need specific exercise programs for sports performance, job demands, and weight management.

You can visit the Elite Physical Therapy Web site (www.elitept1.com) or contact:

Joe Tedesco

Elite Physical Therapy

2630 East Seventh Street, Suite 206

Charlotte, North Carolina 28204